BIRTH MADE EASY

The positive and enjoyable way to have a baby easily and naturally using self-hypnosis

Inner Power Hypnobirthing and the Miracle of Life

Paola Bagnall

www.innerpowerhypnobirthing.co.uk

www.innerpower.co.uk

Birth Made Easy - The positive and enjoyable way to have a baby easily and naturally using self-hypnosis

©Paola Bagnall

ISBN: 978-1-906316-87-7

Published in 2011 by HotHive Books, Evesham, UK.
www.thehothive.com

Disclaimer
A number of complex factors influence the outcome of any self-help strategy. While benefits are typically observed in the majority of cases, there can be no guarantee of success.

The information, ideas and suggestions in this book are intended as an addition to, rather than a substitute for, professional medical advice.

This book is dedicated to my two wonderful sons,
David and Andrew,
who have given me immense joy
and are continuing to do so.

ACKNOWLEDGEMENTS

I would like to thank everyone who has supported me in writing this book. Thank you for making my dream of giving mothers a positive outlook on birth a reality.

I would like to thank the mothers who have used this technique so successfully and given their positive feedback.

I would like to thank Briony Horkan for the great photo she took of me on the back cover.

I also thank Anthony and Renée Hasseldine for the use of their very happy photo on the front cover. This photo was taken by Renée Callander.

My special thanks go to Emma Johnson, who has kept me going through each chapter with her ongoing encouragement and enthusiasm, and to my son David for all the drawings, which are wonderful.

Paola Bagnall's method is revolutionary. It transformed my feelings about my second pregnancy from dread to joyful anticipation and gave me a wonderful natural childbirth.

Her empowering approach gives control of the birth process back to women, and minimises the need for medical intervention and pain relief.

The book's clear and gentle style makes for an easy and enjoyable read, making it accessible to all. The CD's hypnotic routine is powerful and immediately inspirational. If you are nervous about your pregnancy, birth or ability as a new mother, allow Paola Bagnall to change your mind.

Emma Johnson – a hypnobirthing mum

Birth Made Easy by Paola Bagnall is a comprehensive and lucid guide for all pregnant women who aim to have a natural birth with a minimum of medical intervention. The book covers all stages of pregnancy from a biological, psychological and emotional perspective, including the postnatal phase. Throughout the book, the reader can find clear and easy-to-follow diagrams.

The book starts with a useful introduction to the practice and history of hypnotherapy, a form of meditation and relaxation, which works in unison with the healing forces of the unconscious. The use of the technique of hypnotherapy in childbirth is just one of its manifold beneficial applications.

The book, together with a CD, enables the reader to teach herself the art of self-hypnosis by freeing the powers of the unconscious mind. The predominant aim is the preparation for a birth in which self-hypnosis is the main means of pain relief. As one of the first mothers who were prepared by Paola Bagnall for a birth without any invasive pain relief, I can say that it worked amazingly well. I have no memory of pain but only that of a very enjoyable event. The book cites a variety of mothers who had positive experiences with hypnobirthing and who are happy to share their ways of making it work for them.

I have, ever since, recommended self-hypnosis to other prospective mothers. The technique, once learned, will help in all other areas of life and for some becomes an integral part of life after giving birth.

Juliane Horn – a hypnobirthing mum

In this modern technology-driven age it's a relief to have straightforward, practical and reassuring advice on childbirth, and it works! I am so grateful to Paola Bagnall and her techniques for helping me to experience two wonderful and natural births.

Paola sets out clearly how to prepare for childbirth and allows expectant mums to enjoy and focus on pregnancy in a positive way. As a biologist, she's expert in the science of childbirth too, so she provides clear and reassuring explanations of what's happening to your body.

The book is written in Paola's relaxed and warm style, so you can easily learn the techniques to keep yourself calm, reduce pain and maintain some control over your body. This book is essential reading for any expectant mothers – nervous or otherwise – to allow them to have the wonderful childbirth experience they deserve. I can't recommend it enough.

Sarah Findell – a hypnobirthing mum

ANT AND RENÉE HASSELDINE'S STORY

The photo on the front cover is of my cousins Ant and Renée Hasseldine who live in Melbourne, Australia. I think it is a wonderful picture of happiness.

Renée has a bicornuate uterus, which means that the upper part is bifurcated (heart-shaped). This has created a problem for her in sustaining a pregnancy to full term and as a result she has unfortunately experienced two early miscarriages.

As soon as Renée discovered for the first time that she was pregnant, I sent her an inner power hypnobirthing CD. Because she had been listening to that a great deal she was familiar before the miscarriage with the relaxation techniques and the use of colours for healing. We had also spoken a few times via Skype so that I could explain more fully what she needed to do to maintain her self-hypnosis.

Renée sought my help when the miscarriage occurred because she was experiencing severe pain as a result of her uterus contracting very strongly to excrete the foetus. She also wanted to avoid a D&C (surgical removal of the lining and contents of the uterus), as with her uterine structure the foetus quite often does not come away completely and infection can follow. I was able to explain to her how to use self-hypnosis and healing in her situation so that she became calm. She allowed her body to do its work, the miscarriage occurred naturally and in the end she did not need any medical intervention. When the second miscarriage occurred, she coped very well from the start as she knew exactly what to do.

Just a few months later Renée was pregnant again and she used the hypnobirthing techniques to keep her calm throughout the pregnancy. As each week passed, Renée was more certain that this time she would go to term – and she did. Unfortunately, her baby was then very comfortable where she was and an induction had to be carried out 14 days past her due date.

Renée had a needle phobia and was more apprehensive about the induction needle and drip than the birth. With my guidance, her husband Ant recorded a guided visualisation for her (very similar to the one in Chapter Three), which she played while the doctor was hooking up the drip. This took a while, as her veins are a bit tricky and he had a bit of trouble poking and prodding around, but they asked the doctor not to speak to her, and with the assistance of the hypnobirthing techniques she was fine because she managed to dissociate from the hospital and what was going on around her.

Renée had a completely natural birth which she enjoyed. Their daughter, Callista, eventually arrived safely and happily and her parents adore her.

CONTENTS

LIST OF DRAWINGS

CD TRACKS

Track 1 Precautions – where and how to listen to the CD

Track 2 The hypnobirthing programme

Track 3 Background music to the hypnobirthing programme

This can be played during the birth process to keep you calm, relaxed and in control as it will act as a trigger for the birth programme.

It can also be used after the birth of the baby to soothe your baby if it is restless, as your baby will have been listening to the CD along with you before it was born.

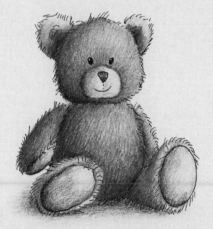

FOREWORD

"Where your focus goes your energy flows."

You are embarking on a most wonderful and magical experience. You are creating a bond like no other, and an experience that will live in your memory for ever.

A rollercoaster of emotions awaits you. It is one of the most emotional times you are likely to encounter. In fact the word 'e-motion' describes a set of feelings which are moving. You can be carried along by this array of emotions, perhaps overwhelmed by them at times; or you can choose to take control of the flow. This book can help you make this time one that you will treasure for the rest of your life.

The miracle of life and the feeling of first holding your baby in your arms cannot be described. You need to *experience* it to fully understand it.

In my 14 years' experience of using hypnotherapy, it has never ceased to amaze me how useful and important hypnosis and self-hypnosis continue to be. Hypnosis has proved itself as a method for transforming people, so they can achieve whatever it is that they need to do. The saying "where your focus goes your energy flows" has never been more important than in childbirth. You can make the whole process a wonderful experience by building up your own self-confidence and self-belief.

The breathing techniques in this book are invaluable. The different self-hypnosis scripts can be used by anyone, no matter what their experience. The CD works effectively and efficiently. This book will help you to acquire important skills, not just for childbirth, but for life.

This book can be used both as a tool for mothers giving birth, and as an invaluable assistance to those in the medical and psychological professions.

Elliott Wald
(Hypnosis expert, television and media hypnotist, author)

I am a biology teacher, having taught in a comprehensive school and then in a sixth-form college. In 1998, I injured my right shoulder by overstretching when decorating the nine-foot high walls in my home. I was in considerable pain. Having had four cortisone injections, osteopathy and physiotherapy the medical profession said to me, "Well, what do you expect at your age?" I was just 50 years young and felt mortified that I was now considered to be old and past it. X-rays had shown I had damaged the soft tissue around the shoulder joint, the tendons and ligaments, which caused the muscles to spasm and increase my pain. I certainly was not going to give up and accept that I now had to live with this problem for the rest of my life.

I could no longer use the whiteboards at school as I could not raise my arm to reach them. So I had to be provided with an overhead projector in each classroom I taught in. (These were the days before the interactive whiteboards linked to a laptop computer.)

In 1999, an acquaintance told me about self-hypnosis, which she had recently discovered. With her encouragement I went on a workshop. This totally changed my life.

I discovered the innate ability we all have to heal ourselves, if we desire to, by harnessing the inner power of the mind. My shoulder healed quickly and I have restored full mobility. So it is now as it was. I did indeed heal myself.

Having discovered this amazing tool, I felt I had to learn more. I enrolled on a hypnotherapy course for 15 months. The more I learnt, the more fascinated I became. I wanted to tell the world of the remarkable inner power we all have.

I qualified as a hypnotherapist in 2000. I continued teaching, and while I was at school I gave the staff and students relaxation classes. Relaxation is natural hypnosis. The staff found they were calmer and could cope with all the pressures of teaching. The students improved their revision, memory and exam successes too. I gave the students a recording to help them, and many used this right through university to keep calm during their revision and exams, to achieve their full potential.

After four years, I had so many clients I decided that I could no longer do both jobs. So after 35 years of teaching, I made the traumatic decision to retire from a job I truly loved, to concentrate on helping people to heal themselves.

I have helped many people to deal with illness and lead better lives. With hypnosis you can have better quality sleep, learn to relax and manage stress, improve confidence and self-esteem, improve relationships, become a better public speaker, improve memory and pass exams easily, reduce weight, become a non-smoker, overcome phobias, and so much more. Hypnosis can be used to improve almost anything in your life.

Hypnosis is very effective in controlling pain, and so, due to my knowledge of the human body, I have specialised in helping mums-to-be to have a natural childbirth.

I feel honoured to have helped so many people to improve their lives and experiences by teaching them the power of hypnosis.

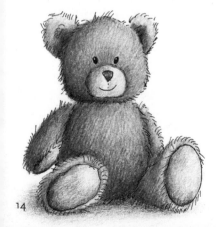

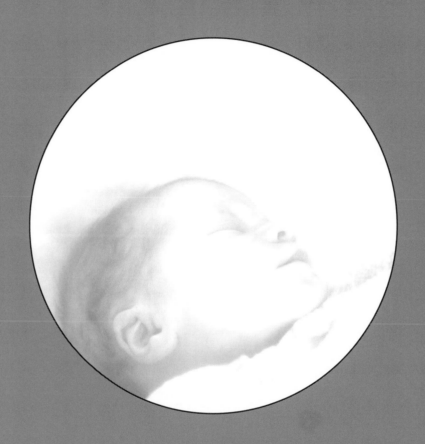

INTRODUCTION

The female body is designed biologically to give birth. Reading this book and using the accompanying CD will reassure you that having a natural birth is well within your capabilities.

You can be in control. You can enjoy your pregnancy. You can look forward to the birth with excitement and anticipation and feel positive and confident about it.

Sometimes medical intervention may be necessary to ensure the health of you and your baby, and this advice should be adhered to. The information, ideas and suggestions in this book are intended as additions to professional advice. However, the methods suggested in this book can also help you to be calm, relaxed and in control during any necessary procedure.

However in many cases a natural childbirth is possible without medical intervention. Trust the power of your body. You want to be in control of the birth, with your baby in the correct position and born very close to your due date. Self-hypnosis can help you with all these things.

Self-hypnosis can help you bond easily with your baby. It can help you to breastfeed if you choose to do so.

It can help you to heal up after the birth, to feel happy and full of energy and able to cope with everything you need to do.

It can help you to get your figure back to pre-pregnancy size, shape and weight very soon after the birth.

All you have to do is to use your self-hypnosis, want it to work and believe it is going to work, and it just does.

Trust your intuition and instincts. You can be a wonderful mother.

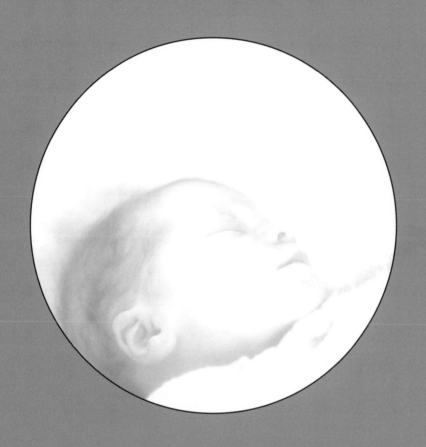

CHAPTER ONE:
ABOUT HYPNOSIS

Historically, hypnosis has been associated with sleep and loss of consciousness. Hypnosis is restful and relaxing but it is not the same as slumber. Brainwave researchers compare hypnosis to the alpha-theta state, which is also similar to that experienced in meditation.

When you are in hypnosis you are aware of your surroundings (sounds, smells, and movements around you) and you are also in control of your actions. Consciousness is not lost. It just becomes more selective. In hypnosis it is usual to be more aware of your internal processes than of what is going on in the world around you. In this altered state, you can select what you want to be aware of, such as concentrating on solving a problem, controlling pain or just enjoying the relaxation.

When a suggestion is given in hypnosis, it penetrates deeply into your unconscious mind, so that it can re-programme your conscious mind for the better. Hypnosis helps your unconscious resources to change your behaviour. This is powerful because the mind can control/change/improve almost anything that it wants to by communicating with the unconscious mind. Hypnosis frees you from the constraints of your conscious mind, allowing you to move from analysis and rigid thinking to the imaginative and creative resources of the unconscious.

Each person is unique, and everyone experiences hypnosis differently. However, basically, hypnosis is entering an 'altered state'. Hypnosis involves no loss of mental control. It is simply a way of getting directly into the unconscious mind.

In hypnosis, your breathing rate and heart beat will slow down, the bronchi of your lungs will dilate, your blood pressure will drop and the production of your stomach acid will reduce. No stress hormones will be released into the bloodstream. Your white blood cells will cling more firmly to your blood vessels, which may increase your body's immune efficiency. This 'altered state' of deep relaxation helps you to contact your unconscious mind, bringing 'inner power' to promote desired changes and physical well-being.

In fact, everyone experiences hypnosis regularly. This is natural hypnosis and occurs 60 per cent of the day for most people. It occurs just before you fall asleep and just as you awake. Other examples include when you have lost track of time when reading a good book or watching something interesting on television. It can even occur while driving, when you arrive at your destination and do not know how you got there. In essence, hypnosis is simply a state of heightened relaxation and altered awareness.

When you are relaxed in this way it is possible to make contact with your unconscious mind, in order to effect change in your life. The unconscious is an untapped resource for creativity.

The unconscious mind is the seat of all your emotions and so directs nearly all your behaviour. Most importantly, your unconscious is responsible for maintaining your body in good health and for all the autonomic processes – for example, breathing, blood circulation, tissue repair and controlling blood sugar level.

Hypnosis is a doorway to the realms of your imagination and emotions, your 'inner power'. Using hypnosis, the unconscious mind can be contacted. This 'inner power' can be harnessed to promote desired changes and physical well-being, and this can help you in childbirth.

The conscious mind (or left brain) processes information logically and linearly, literally in a straight line (1, 2, 3, 4, 5, etc). It is rational and organised, often referred to as the 'analytical mind'. The left brain also controls our voluntary (somatic) nervous system.

The unconscious mind (or right brain) on the other hand, sees relationships in information and processes them in random, abstract patterns; even when pieces to the answer are missing. The right brain is creative, intuitive, irrational and emotional. The right brain controls our involuntary (autonomic) nervous system. Through ideo-motor responses (physical movements or behaviour in response to an idea or thought in the mind), we can speed up or slow down our heart, and even alter the chemical balance in our body to fight off disease. A mother giving birth could secrete more serotonins to create the body's natural epidural. The unconscious mind, therefore, runs our bodies for us, controlling all the automatic processes of nervous and hormonal control. It is the home of our emotions, creativity, imagination and all our memories.

The two sides of our brain communicate with each other constantly mixing logical, rational thoughts with the abstract and emotional.

Many authorities believe the unconscious uses 90 per cent of the brain capacity and that from birth (possibly even while in the womb) it has been recording everything that happens to us. We use our conscious minds to analyse events and make decisions (when they are based on logic rather than insight or feelings). The mind, then, is like an iceberg. The conscious mind is the 10 per cent which sticks up above the water. It helps us with daily decision-making processes and also assists us in new situations where we apply rational thinking to fathom out what to do and how to do it. The unconscious mind is the hidden depths of the iceberg (the 90 per cent submerged below the water) and works on 'auto-pilot', dealing with a variety of tasks, such as the emotions, imagination, memories and the autonomic nervous system.

In another metaphor which illustrates the relationship between the conscious and unconscious mind, the unconscious mind is represented by a dark room. If you enter the room with a torch (representing the conscious mind) you can pick out details of the room, and focus on only a few things at a time. The rest of the room is there, but you cannot see it, just as you cannot see the unconscious mind.

The conscious mind remembers only a part of what the entire mind has learned and experienced throughout life. However, the unconscious mind remembers everything.

The conscious mind often represses what lies in the unconscious mind, and these events can often only be recalled by a stimulus (such as a particular perfume, or picture) which links us to a past memory.

It is interesting to know that the unconscious mind has no concept of time. So, for example, something that happened at five years of age may still feel as though it is happening now, with the same intensity, just as it did then. This can happen when a mother has had a difficult birth. However, the conscious mind does have a concept of time, and through hypnosis this time distortion can be rectified and the 'event' re-framed and put into its correct perspective.

Hypnosis is therefore an altered state of consciousness, in which you can manifest heightened suggestibility and selective thought. Through hypnosis, you can tap into the 'inner power' of your mind. You can by-pass the critical evaluating facilities of your conscious mind, and penetrate your unconscious mind. In this way, you can help your body to achieve a wonderful experience of childbirth.

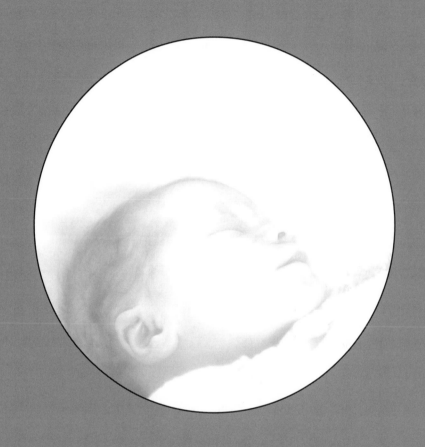

CHAPTER TWO:
PREGNANCY, BIRTH AND AFTER
THE BIRTH: HYPNOBIRTHING

You may be constantly bombarded with negative stories about childbirth.

You may have been told that it is the most painful thing you will ever do in your life. You may have heard all the gory details of births that had complications and all the medical intervention that could occur.

All this often makes some of us feel a bit anxious and worried about childbirth. It is no wonder that some mothers feel tense and unable to relax in childbirth. It is no wonder that the 'pain' of childbirth then becomes a reality. Hypnosis can help you to put all this into perspective.

Childbirth is a natural process. It is one that women's bodies were designed for. When you are calm and relaxed, your muscles and skin stretch easily and naturally in a pain-free way. When you are happy, you will have more confidence in your own abilities as a mother.

Hypnobirthing is a philosophy and technique for achieving a satisfying, relaxing and stress-free birth. It teaches you to call on your body's own natural epidural, which can help to eliminate the need for medication. This allows your body and your baby to work together in the most natural way possible. You stay focused on the process and are in tune with what your body and intuition are telling you.

Hypnobirthing mothers are totally aware and fully in control as they bring their babies into the world. As a result of this, giving birth becomes an exciting and pleasurable experience, just as it should be.

Using self-hypnosis for childbirth can help you:

- ★ put things into perspective, so that you enjoy your pregnancy and have a wonderful childbirth
- ★ relax and be calm and in control
- ★ stay focused and be in tune with what your body is telling you
- ★ become healthier and fitter
- ★ control or reduce pain without drugs
- ★ promote rapid healing and recovery
- ★ enjoy better quality sleep
- ★ breastfeed naturally
- ★ heal up quickly after the birth
- ★ reduce weight after the birth easily
- ★ improve your confidence as a mother

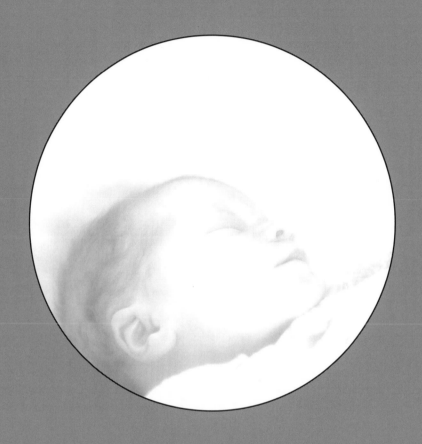

CHAPTER THREE:
VISUALISATION SCRIPT FOR
SELF-HYPNOSIS

This chapter gives you a relaxation technique (which is self-hypnosis) and should be practised as often as possible before the baby's due date, preferably daily. When you are having contractions, you can use this technique to take you to a special place and really feel that you are there. You can also use a colour to relax, and imagine that it flows over you, helping you to remain in control of your baby's birth. Daydreaming techniques like this help you to dissociate yourself from the 'feelings' of the contractions.

The subconscious mind cannot tell the difference between what is real and unreal. So when you really imagine that you are in your favourite place, then your unconscious mind will think that you are actually there, and respond by secreting lots of serotonins (the 'happy' hormone as I call it), so you feel good about yourself. Using this relaxation technique during the birth process produces a natural epidural to help you cope with the contractions.

The easiest way of doing this relaxation daily is to:

- ★ make a recording of the script that follows
- ★ choose your special place and your colour of relaxation (you do not need all of them)
- ★ sit in a comfortable chair or lie down
- ★ just listen to the words (without having to think about them!)

Your birth partner is a very important part of the process of hypnobirthing. When you do this relaxation for the first time, get your birth partner to read out the script to you, so you can allow your unconscious to select your special place and a colour. Then when you make the recording, you can just describe your own special place and your colour (or colours). If you have the technology, you can record your voice (or your birth partner's voice) with gentle relaxing music in the background.

The CD that goes with this book takes you through a much shorter version of the relaxation script, and will help you to find *your* special place and *your* colour (or colours). However, by making your own recording, you can make it more personal, by describing your own special place and colour (or colours), and also ensure that your partner is familiar with this too.

It is not essential to make your own recording, as the CD helps you to do this in your mind's eye. The following script will help you understand the process and it will also help your partner know what to say to you during the contractions.

The script for relaxation and self-hypnosis

Sit in a comfortable chair or lie down. Cover yourself with a blanket to ensure you are warm, as when you relax deeply your metabolic rate lowers and you can feel a bit chilly.

Take five deep breaths. Breathe in to a count of four and out to a count of six.

And in your mind you may choose to imagine yourself being somewhere where you can really relax: a place to take it easy and be comfortable, calm and at ease, maybe a beach, a favourite place or somewhere you have always wanted to go, somewhere you can relax more and more and more. Somewhere for you to go, knowing there is nothing you have to do. This is an opportunity for you to be away from, separated from, the outside world for a little while at least to spend some time within, to spend some time deeper and deeper down, relaxing more and more, letting go more and more with each and every gentle and relaxed breath you take.

With each breath that you breathe in you have a wonderful sense of well-being. With each breath you breathe out you relax more and more.

And in your mind you may like to imagine yourself on a beach, a wonderful sandy beach in a cove, surrounded by mountains. And as you feel the wonderful warm sun on your body you relax more. As you lie on the sand the cries of the gulls soaring into the sky take you deeper and deeper. The smell and sounds of the sea as it runs up the shore relax your body and relax your mind taking you deeper and deeper into relaxation. Each and every feeling allows you to relax more and more easily, comfortably.

Maybe you can imagine yourself walking through a woodland on a bright spring day and as you see the sun's rays gently and easily glistening through the leaves creating a dappled carpet of light, you relax more and more knowing that there is nothing you have to do. Each and every step you take, takes you deeper and deeper down, more and more relaxed. The rustling of the leaves and the fresh, cool breeze against your face, the beautiful spring flowers, the glow of the bluebells, all promise a fresh start, as the continuous unbroken continuity of nature is like magic taking you deeper and deeper down, so calm, relaxed, at ease.

Maybe you can imagine yourself in a field in late summer full of dandelion 'clocks'. A sudden gust of wind blows the parachute seeds high into the air and then they gently and easily drift down and down floating on the air currents, and as they fall to the ground you go deeper and deeper down, more and more relaxed.

Maybe you can experience yourself sitting in a meadow full of daisies by the side of a stream hearing the water running over the stones so you drift further and further into a wonderful deep relaxation.

Choose somewhere, be somewhere where you can relax and let go; somewhere that is comfortable and calm for you to be; somewhere where you can leave the world behind for a little while at least; somewhere where you can be comfortable and calm, relaxed and at ease.

Maybe whatever you chose to lie on, or sit on, for this relaxation session now feels as though it is becoming softer and softer and your head is sinking a little more into the pillow, or whatever your head is lying on. You feel and are more and more comfortable, more and more relaxed, more and more at ease.

And each and every thought, every feeling, every emotion is taking you deeper and deeper down, relaxing you more and more.

Maybe you can imagine yourself at the top of a mountain with crisp white snow, and as you ski down and down, gathering momentum, you relax more and more easily.

Maybe you are in a deep warm bath, wallowing in soapy bubbles. The water is at just the right temperature, a comfortable, relaxed, easy feeling as you relax more and more and more, going deeper and deeper, letting go.

Or maybe you are deep sea diving among the tropical fish, all shapes and sizes and colours. You swim with them deeper and deeper down, and you relax more and more, a comfortable easy feeling of deep relaxation.

Choose somewhere of your liking. Imagine somewhere you really want to be; somewhere where you feel, and are, happy, carefree; where you can be alone and relax; somewhere you can let go, drifting deeper and deeper into relaxation.

And notice quite how wonderfully relaxed your body is feeling and being. Maybe you can imagine this deep relaxation as a beautiful crystal blue colour, or a turquoise green or even a yellow. Choose a colour of relaxation for you. It could be red or orange, pink or purple, white or cream. Sometimes the unconscious mind likes to choose more than one colour and that is OK too.

Feel, visualise this colour spreading easily and naturally from your eyelids over your forehead and to the back of your head releasing any tension you may feel. The colour spreads round to your cheeks and down to your jaws. The colour relaxes each and every muscle as it passes over you. You are now so relaxed that you may feel your lower jaw fall a little lower than usual as you are relaxing progressively more and more.

The colour spreads to your chin and down your neck to your shoulders, relaxing and releasing any stress you may feel, any tightness in the muscles. The colour relaxes every part of you in turn enabling you to relax even further, and so you do.

The colour spreads down your arms, to your elbows and into your hands, relaxing every muscle, every fibre, tendon and joint reaching your fingers and thumbs, and as the colour reaches your fingertips you may notice a tingling sensation, a momentary feeling as you relax more and more, going deeper and deeper into relaxation. A comfortable experience, a pleasant feeling that tells you, you are even more relaxed.

The colour now glides to your chest and down to your tummy, round your navel and to your lower abdomen. The colour relaxes every muscle, tendon, ligament, joint, each and every cell, molecule and atom is relaxing, being at ease.

The colour you have chosen promotes a better balance in every part of you, better harmony, so all your internal organs support each other and work in unison for your well-being. You feel, and are, even more and more relaxed.

The warmth of the colour spreads round to your back relaxing each and every muscle. It moves down to your hips and buttocks and glides over your thighs to your knees and down your shins and to your calves reaching your ankles, relaxing you more and more. So this deep relaxation is spreading through your body and finally it reaches your feet and your toes where it may create another momentary tingling feeling at the tips of your toes. A pleasant feeling, a momentary experience, a comfortable experience that tells you, you are more and more relaxed. Your entire body is at peace, tranquil, so calm and relaxed.

This colour that you have chosen now totally surrounds you with deep relaxation, surrounding you with love, linking you into the universal energy of life so that you have all the energy you require to have a wonderfully natural childbirth. And so you do have a wonderfully natural childbirth.

By being relaxed you work with your body so childbirth is a pleasant, exciting experience for you.

And now as you count from one to five you are coming out of this deep relaxation feeling and being relaxed, calm and in control.

1, 2, 3, 4 and 5. (It is advisable to count fairly slowly.)

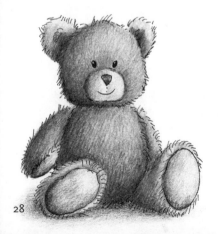

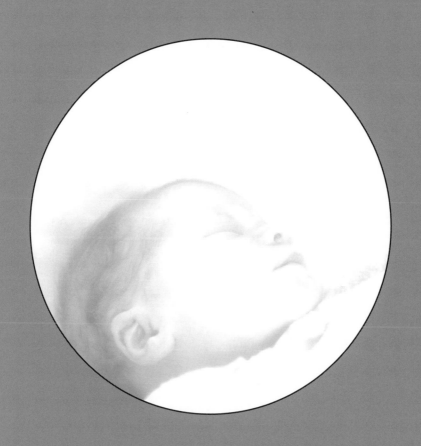

CHAPTER FOUR:
BIRTH IMAGES

You may want to visualise yourself giving birth. Visualising the experience will help you to rehearse child-birthing in a positive, relaxing way.

If you practise self-hypnosis regularly, you will develop some post-hypnotic cues which will give you the feeling of comfort and relaxation at the times you need them during the birth process.

When you are relaxed, you allow your body to open up easily, naturally and quickly during the first stage, so you can be in control of your baby's birth.

Below are some suggestions that you may like to use. They are suggestions of images given to me by mothers who have worked with me when going through childbirth.

"I imagined my delivery as rose petals opening and unfolding to reveal a lovely new baby. With each deep breath I saw myself as that rose blossoming."

Flowers are a very good image to use, as you can imagine a tight bud opening up into a beautiful bloom. You can be very precise about the colour and type of flower you use. Choose one that means something to you personally. For example, a lotus flower bud opening, or a magnolia flower opening.

As you see the flower bud opening up more and more, so you allow your body to relax and work as it should do, opening up to allow your baby to be born easily and naturally.

Using a beach image and the sounds of the waves can be very effective also.

"I used self-hypnosis for the birth of my two children. I made a self-hypnosis CD and listened to it daily in the weeks before the deliveries so I was able to relax my body parts individually and in groups. While in a trance, I imagined a warm, sunny walk at a beautiful sandy beach with seagulls and a soft wind blowing my hair. I became aware of my breathing and I visualised that with each rise and fall of the contractions my cervix was opening more and more like a flower opening. It helped me create a positive, controlled, and aware understanding of a wonderful experience."

"I used the image of waves crashing against the rocks and as the waves subsided so I relaxed more and more and my body opened up more and more."

"I used the image of waves rolling up my favourite beach. As the waves flowed gently up the shore this was the height of the contraction. As the water flowed back to the sea, so I allowed my body to relax and to open up easily and naturally."

Flowers and beaches and waves are the most popular of the birth images. However, many other images have been used by my hypnobirthing mums.

"The more intense the contractions became, the more I rubbed my stomach. I pictured each breath I took as a rush of new life going in my nose and down to the baby. As I breathed deeper, I felt that this was also bringing more relaxation and calm to me and to my child. I had gone over this picture many times while I was in a trance in the weeks before my labour."

"I visualised my uterus as an upside down sea anemone without any tentacles and with each contraction the mouth of the sea anemone got bigger and bigger and so my body opened up more and more."

"A swing in the garden, swinging up to a crescendo with the contractions and then releasing and swinging back down as the contraction subsided, so allowing my body to open up more and more."

"I saw rings of colour in the shape of a flower, and with each contraction the rings of colour would move down and get bigger and bigger, so allowing me to relax more and more and my body to open up easily, naturally."

"I really enjoy playing tennis, so I imagined playing a hard game of tennis and this allowed me to relax and just let my cervix open up naturally, and as I was so relaxed I was able to let my uterus do the work it needed to."

"I love running marathons and so I imagined myself running a race and remaining focused on the running and so allowing my body to open up easily because I was so relaxed, focused and in control."

"I imagined throwing a pebble into a pond and the ripples getting larger and larger. As this happened so my body opened up more and more."

"I saw myself climbing up a hill as the contractions began, and then running down the other side as the contraction eased off." (This in fact describes the graph of the perfect contraction as shown in Chapter Eight.)

Be as creative as you want to be in developing your own images and post-hypnotic cues. These cues could be rubbing your abdomen or holding your partner's hand, and these can then help you achieve more comfort and calm.

It can be fun making your own self-hypnosis and relaxation techniques. It will also be very helpful when you go through childbirth as it will seem all the more personal.

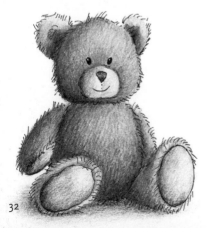

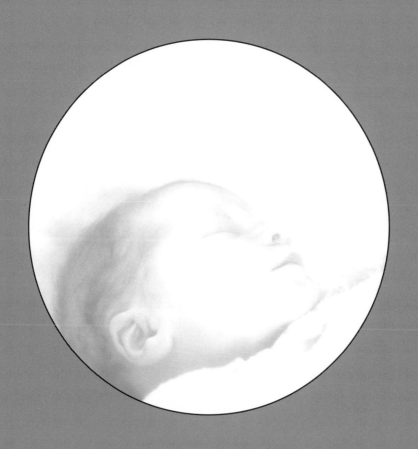

CHAPTER FIVE:
USING THE BREATH

Fear, shock or stress can make us panic. Your body responds to panic by producing the hormone adrenalin.

The hormone adrenalin produces dramatic changes in the body. It prepares your body for swift action, and so is also called the 'fright, fight and flight' hormone.

Adrenalin causes an increase in the rate of the heart beat and heart output, the ventilation rate, and the constriction of small blood vessels in the skin and abdomen, so more blood circulates to the skeletal muscles, taking more oxygen and sugars. The general effect is that the whole body is ready for vigorous action, which might be necessary in an emergency.

As the blood is taken away from the digestive system so more goes to the muscles creating the 'butterflies in the tummy' effect. In extreme cases this can cause the voiding of the bladder and bowels.

This state of tension cannot be tolerated for long periods and usually other hormones destroy the adrenalin.

When you feel fear, adrenalin is produced in large quantities. The more fear you feel, then the more adrenalin is produced.

So to counteract the adrenalin production, concentrating on breathing automatically reduces its flow as it reduces our fear.

Breathing technique one

Breathe in to a count of four.
Breathe out to a count of six.
Repeat this as many times as required, and at least fifteen times.

This sends a signal to the unconscious mind to reduce the adrenalin flow. In this way you are always in control.

Breathing technique two: the programme for three deeper breaths

★   Breath 1 brings instant mental calmness.
    As you breathe out SAY to yourself, "I am calm".

★ Breath 2 brings instant feelings of physical relaxation.
   As you breathe out SAY to yourself, "I am relaxed".
★ Breath 3 brings instant feelings of confidence.
   As you breathe out SAY to yourself "I am confident"
                                             "I can do ..."

Breathing technique two can be used whenever you want instant feelings of calmness, relaxation and confidence. Using the breath reduces the adrenalin flow, so creating calmness and relaxation.

I find it easier to say a few words after each breath, as it keeps me focused on what I am doing. (Suggestions of what you can say after each breath are given above, but you can use your own words.)

You can use this breathing programme in any situation where more calmness, relaxation and confidence are required. It is not just for being pregnant or for the birth of the baby. It can be used at work, rest or play!

Positive affirmations

In breathing technique two, at breath 3, you are using positive affirmations. An affirmation is anything you say or think and this affects your unconscious mind. In fact, your thinking determines a great deal. Think negatively, and you attract negative realities. Think positively, and the benefits you desire in life may well come true.

Say your affirmation in the present tense, as if it is happening now. Say what you want to happen. For pregnancy and birth, the list of affirmations is endless:

"I enjoy my pregnancy."
"My digestive system works efficiently and effectively."
"My digestive system is more and more comfortable." (This is used to overcome early morning sickness.)
"I look forward to the birth with excitement."
"I have a wonderfully natural childbirth."
"I heal up easily after the birth."
"I breastfeed easily."
"I enjoy being a mum."
"I trust my instincts and intuition."

"I am a wonderful mother."
"When I feel tired I rest for half an hour and listen to track 3 on Paola's CD."
"I have all the energy I need."
"I am doing great."
"I am doing fantastically well."

Use your imagination and you can make up as many affirmations as you wish.

Émile Coué (1857–1926) put forward the 'Law of Concentrated Attention', which states, "Whenever attention is concentrated on an idea over and over again, it spontaneously tends to realise it."

Therefore keep on saying your affirmations and they will spontaneously happen for you. You can use them when things are going well. You can also use them when things have gone wrong and you need to redirect yourself, and things really will get better.

Use the programme for the three deeper breaths whenever you can. It will reinforce how you want to feel and be during your pregnancy and during the birth, and afterwards.

This programme can be used in many other ways – for example, to help you deal with a work situation, to improve your sport performance, or to improve relationships with family, friends and work colleagues. The uses are infinite!

Positive affirmations also link up with the 'Law of Attraction', which states that what you put into the universe is reflected back to you. So radiate positivity and calmness, and that is what you get back.

Since the breathing techniques reduce adrenalin they will also help you get back into control if you temporarily lose confidence at any time before, during or after the birth. Breathing technique one is especially good in this situation.

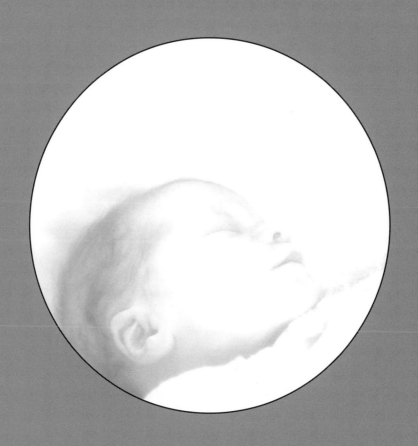

CHAPTER SIX:
THE BIOLOGY OF THE
FEMALE BODY

Now that you are familiar with the process of hypnosis and different methods of breathing, it is important to understand the biology of the female body. When you know about the physical processes of pregnancy and birth, then it is easy to use your self-hypnosis and all the suggested relaxation techniques more effectively.

Fig 6.1 The female reproductive organs

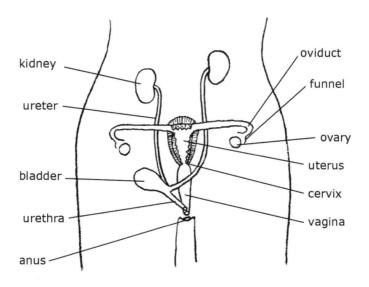

The egg cells called ova are produced in the ovaries and wafted by little hair-like structures (called cilia) into the oviducts (fallopian tubes) where fertilisation may take place.

The production of ova is not continuous throughout life. All the potential egg cells are present in the ovary at birth (roughly 200,000 in each ovary) of which 400 to 500 develop to maturity during the active reproductive life of the female.

The uterus has a thick muscular wall (the myometrium) and a nutritive blood-filled inner lining (the endometrium). This inner lining is the part that helps to make the placenta that provides nutrition for the baby.

Fig 6.2 Side view of the female reproductive organs

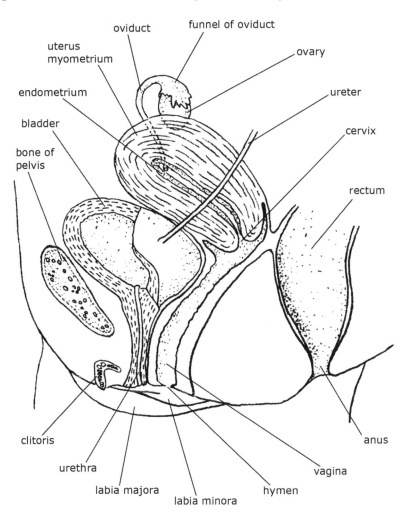

The uterus is made of the same muscle as the digestive system. It is called smooth involuntary muscle, as it is controlled by the unconscious mind.

The lowest part of the uterus and its entrance is called the cervix, which also forms the upper limit to the vagina. The vagina is lined with secreting gland cells, which produce lubricating fluids during sexual arousal. Until puberty, the vagina is partially or almost completely closed by a thin membrane (the hymen), which becomes perforated to allow the menstrual flow.

Surrounding the opening to the vagina are two pairs of fleshy folds (called the labia). The entire region, including the entrances of the urinary and reproductive tracts, is known as the vulva.

At the front of the vulva is the clitoris. This is a small erectile organ similar to the male penis, consisting of spongy tissue and containing nerve endings which heighten sexual arousal on stimulation.

At puberty, usually one ovum from one ovary is released into one of the oviducts every month. This is ovulation. When this starts happening, the female is sexually mature and can produce offspring. If no fertilisation takes place, then the lining of the uterus (the endometrium) is lost, creating the menstrual flow. The uterus lining is then remade ready for the next ovulation.

The act of introducing sperm into the female reproductive tract is sexual intercourse (or coitus). The erect male penis is placed in the vagina and the sperm and seminal fluid are ejaculated by a series of rapid muscular contractions. The force of this sends the sperm right up to the cervix and into the uterus. This creates an orgasm in the male. The female orgasm is usually characterised by contractions of the uterus and vagina. For both partners, the orgasm is the peak of sexual stimulation and is defined as a state of physiological and emotional release associated with extreme pleasure.

Of the 300 million sperm released into the female, only a few thousand reach the oviduct and only a few hundred reach the ovum. Fertilisation therefore depends upon random fusion of the male sperm and female ovum.

When one successful sperm enters the ovum, fertilisation occurs. A zygote is formed by this union, and it is propelled along the oviduct to the uterus by waves of muscular contraction (known as peristalsis). In humans, this process takes a week and then it implants in the uterus.

The motile sperm can move at a rate of one millimetre per minute. They can survive for a few days after entering the female reproductive tract. After ovulation, the ovum lives only for 24 hours. Thus sexual intercourse from about three days before ovulation to one day after ovulation may result in fertilisation. Ovulation usually occurs on day 14 of the 28-day female cycle.

The zygote (fertilised ovum) then divides by a process known as mitosis. By day 3, a mass of 16 cells will have been formed and it is now known as a morula. The morula enters the uterus about one week after fertilisation has occurred. It then becomes a hollow ball of cells with an embryo in the centre, surrounded by three foetal membranes. At this stage the structure is called a blastocyst.

The inner membrane is the amnion and becomes filled with amniotic fluid. This protects the developing baby from knocks, maintains a constant temperature and allows free movement of the baby.

The cavity expands to fill the entire uterus. The two outer membranes unite to form the placenta, which embeds in the endometrium and forms an intimate connection between the embryonic and maternal tissues. The blastocyst starts to implant in the endometrium at about 10 days after fertilisation.

As this occurs, the embryo continues to divide and differentiate, so that all the body parts are formed in the correct places.

Five weeks after implantation, the placenta is well established and is connected by blood vessels to the embryo by means of the umbilical cord.

At the end of two months, all major tissue systems of the embryo are complete. It is 2.5 centimetres long and is now called a foetus.

Gestation is the term for the time from fertilisation until birth.

At 12 weeks, the foetus is fully formed and its sex has been determined. From 13 to 40 weeks is a period of growth.

Normally the uterus is only the size of a clenched fist, and as the baby grows it enlarges to fill the abdominal cavity, so pushing up the digestive system and the diaphragm.

The diagrams on the next page show stages of the embryo developing into the foetus. In the early stages, the embryo could develop into any vertebrate animal – a chicken, a cow or even a chimpanzee – as the stages are very similar. However, by week 8 it can clearly be seen that the foetus is human. This is due to the genetic information contained in the zygote.

Fig 6.3 Stages of the human embryo and foetus

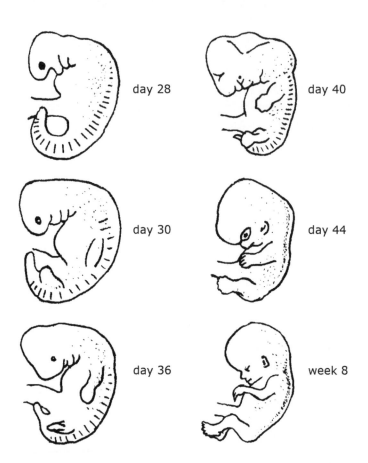

day 28

day 40

day 30

day 44

day 36

week 8

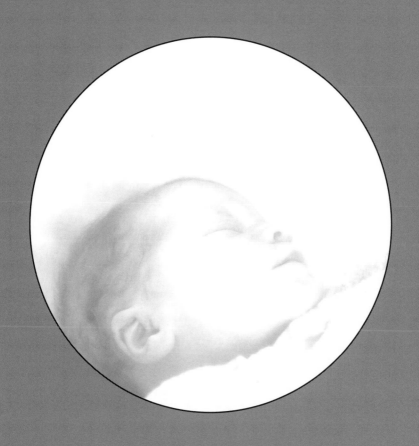

CHAPTER SEVEN:
THE BIOLOGY OF BIRTH

Birth is known as parturition. This is the point of transition between the prenatal and postnatal period of life.

Labour is divided into three stages:

Stage one is the period from the onset of uterine contractions until full dilation of the cervix. This first stage is subdivided into three phases:

★ The Latent or Ripening phase where the cervix softens and dilates from 1–3 centimetres. This stage can take a while and you may not even be aware of it. Sometimes you may experience cramping sensations similar to when you have a period; the mucus plug at the entrance to the cervix may be released or you may possibly get some strong contractions.

★ The Active phase where the cervix dilates from 4–9 centimetres. At this stage the contractions gradually increase in intensity and become much more regular.

★ The Transitional phase where the cervix finally reaches 10 centimetres dilation. Contractions may slow at this stage, as the baby descends further into the birth canal, but not always. Many mothers are not aware of this transitional stage.

Stage two is the time of maximal dilation of the cervix until the baby exits the vagina.

Stage three is the process of expulsion of the placenta through the vagina.

Fig 7.1 Stage one of parturition

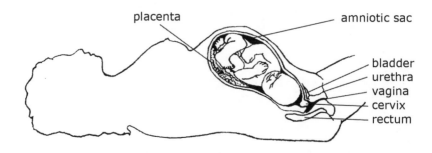

The uterus is made of smooth involuntary muscle. When the time is right for birth this muscle will start contracting, due to a sharp decline in the hormone progesterone and an increase in oestrogen. There is, usually, nothing that will stop it, except medical intervention (if this is deemed necessary).

(For me, personally, feeling the first strong uterine contraction with my first son has been, and will be, the most exciting experience of my life. Perhaps that is because I am a biologist?)

The contractions cause the cervix to dilate to a diameter of 10 centimetres. The increasing pressure placed on the cervix by the baby's head aids this dilation. The contractions are exactly the same sort of contractions that occur in the digestive system (called peristalsis), and are simply waves of contractions followed by a little relaxation. Uterine muscle has the unique ability to contract and retract, which means it remains slightly contracted, thus aiding the process of pushing the baby out and causing further dilation of the cervix.

It is during this phase that hypnosis can help you. When you are relaxed, your body can open up easily, naturally and quickly. There is a mind-body connection, so you can be in control and your body can do its job without any interference. This is achieved because your body responds to relaxation by releasing more serotonins, the happy hormone.

When you lose control and panic (see Chapter Five), the body responds by releasing adrenalin and, unfortunately, more adrenalin creates more panic. When you are calm and relaxed, then the birth can happen more naturally, as it is meant to happen. After all, the female body is designed biologically to give birth. It is during stage one that you can use breathing techniques and visualisations (described in the previous chapters) to ensure the release of serotonins, which are the body's natural pain relief.

It is often at this stage that the amniotic sac ruptures ('breaking of the waters') to create fluid for lubrication for the second stage of birth. The amniotic sac may break at any time during the birth: sometimes before stage one and some babies have even been born in the sac without it breaking! In the latter case the vagina produces the lubrication.

It is important to know that each contraction lasts for only one to one-and-a-half minutes, even with the strongest of contractions. So you need to think of the contractions simply as contractions, rather than as 'pains'. The problem is that if you think 'pain', then pain is what you get. This clearly shows the mind-body connection.

The contractions often start off quite slowly at first and may simply feel like period cramps, especially in the 'Latent' phase. They gradually increase in strength and frequency, so they become much more regular, moving to 15 minutes apart, and then gradually getting to about three minutes apart. This is the time to go to hospital, if you are giving birth there, as this indicates that you have progressed to the 'Active' first stage.

The contractions may be felt either in the lower abdomen, across the entire abdomen, localised in the small of the back or sometimes going down the thighs. They can also be felt in a combination of these places.

Fig 7.2 Stage two of parturition

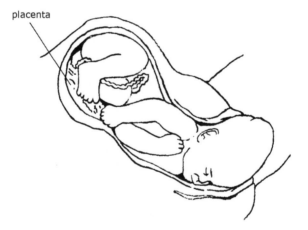

placenta

Stage two is when the cervix is 10 centimetres dilated. The vagina has softened and the perineum is stretching. At this point, with each contraction there is a very strong urge to push.

Hypnosis is not used in the same way at this stage. Now is the time to use all your skeletal muscles, so your abdominal muscles (which are under voluntary control of the brain) are made to contract consciously, to literally push the baby out via the vagina.

It is often said that you need to push as if you are doing a 'poo' the size of a melon. Remember, your uterus works in the same way as the digestive system, using a series of muscular contractions called peristalsis.

Again, each contraction only lasts for one to one-and-a-half minutes. Now you need to push with all your strength to work with your baby and the intuition of your unconscious mind and push strongly only when your body tells you to do so. If you do this, then these contractions are painless (well, they were for me, and the feeling of the baby descending into the vagina was quite wonderful too).

Sometimes there may be a feeling to 'push' before the cervix has reached 10 centimetres dilation. This is because the lip of the cervix has not quite fully stretched. The position of the baby, especially if it is 'back to back' (lying on your back) can also create the urge to push when your body is not quite ready for stage two.

If this occurs then it is crucial that you do not push otherwise the tip of the cervix may swell up. To lessen the strong urge to push, a special breathing technique is used.

Breathing technique for the no pushing stage

Simply pant, like a dog, with the mouth open, breathing in and out through the mouth, with the tongue resting on the lower lip. Continue doing this for the one to one-and-a-half minutes of the contraction.

Usually stage one (the opening and widening stage) is smoothly followed by stage two (the pushing stage). Once the head is out of the vagina, it will rotate naturally and on its own, and then it takes just one more contraction and the baby is born. (A great feeling!) The birth has occurred and a new, beautiful life has entered the world.

It helps if you can get skin-to-skin contact as soon as possible with your baby attached to the umbilical cord. So hold your baby now. You and your baby may be tired after the process of birth, so do not worry if your baby is not ready to start suckling. However, if you can and want to start breastfeeding now, it is a good idea, as it will feel familiar to both of you later on. Putting the baby to the breast also aids delivery of the placenta.

You can then choose to leave the umbilical cord to stop pulsating before it is cut, unless there is a medical reason to protect the baby and you. It is thought that doing this reduces breathing problems in the baby. The cord is clamped before it is cut. Your birth partner can cut the umbilical cord with supervision. This can help them to bond with the baby, too.

Fig 7.3 Stage three of parturition

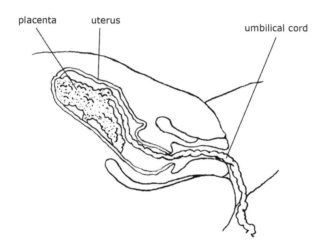

Soon after delivery of the baby, the foetal and maternal blood vessels of the placenta completely contract and the placenta separates from the wall of the uterus by further muscular contractions. This is stage three of the birth and is often called the delivery of the 'afterbirth'. Usually this is hardly noticed, as the placenta is very soft and only weighs between one sixth and one third of the weight of the baby, and the mother is so wrapped up in seeing her baby.

You do have a choice as to the time of the delivery of the placenta. In hospital, it is often advised to have a hormonal injection as soon as the baby is born. This causes the uterus to contract strongly to push out the placenta quickly. Leaving it to happen naturally can take from five minutes to two hours and is usually around 45 minutes. Allowing the process to happen naturally depends on you, and how you feel about allowing everything to occur as naturally as possible. Your midwife will follow your birth plan if you insist, unless there are medical benefits to you, and/or the baby, from the injection. If this is the case the midwife should explain the reasons for this to you.

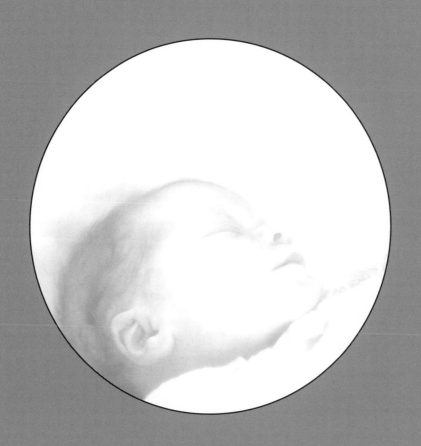

CHAPTER EIGHT:
USING THE CD

The CD with this book takes you through all the stages: the pregnancy, the three stages of the birth itself, healing up after the birth, bonding with your baby, breastfeeding, getting your figure back to pre-pregnancy weight, size and shape and being confident as a mother.

Start listening to the CD as soon as you can. The earlier in your pregnancy you listen to the CD the better. However, it is beneficial at any stage. The more you hear the CD, the more your unconscious mind knows what to do during the birth.

All you have to do is make sure you are in a safe, quiet place, somewhere you can completely relax. So choose a comfortable place, where you can be sitting or lying down.

This CD is not to be used when you are driving or doing anything that requires your concentration, or if you suffer from epilepsy. You can use your CD with earphones if you are a passenger. However, the best place is to be in a situation where you are not going to be disturbed for the duration of the CD.

When in hypnosis and the alpha-theta brainwave pattern you can feel a bit chilly, so it is advisable to cover yourself with a blanket to ensure you are warm. This is because the metabolic rate of the body lowers during relaxation and hypnosis.

When you play the CD, allow your eyes to close, and as you listen you automatically go into hypnosis. You may notice that you start to feel light and floaty, or really heavy, as if you cannot be bothered to move. Some people feel both light and heavy at the same time. You may notice a fluttering in the eyelids. Others get loud tummy rumblings. Whatever you experience in hypnosis is the correct feeling for you, and it is always a very comfortable feeling. Some people notice very little difference at first.

A point to note is that, while playing the CD, you do not have to concentrate on every word. Your mind is free to wander. You can think your own thoughts because your unconscious mind is so powerful, it can listen to and hear the words on the CD while your conscious mind is thinking about other things.

Listening to the CD is a bit like putting a program into a computer. However, with the unconscious mind, the repetition means that you are calm throughout the pregnancy. When the waters break, or the contractions start, then the CD programme automatically goes into effect for the birth without you listening to the CD at this stage. (This is a trigger that I have put into the CD programme, so it takes effect as soon as you start the birth process.)

By listening to the CD early on in the pregnancy, you will have chosen your special place already. I give a few suggestions on the CD and your unconscious mind chooses the best place for you, which could be quite different from my suggestions. This is the same for your colours of relaxation. I make a few suggestions and then you choose the ones that are right for you (see Chapter Three). You will also have chosen your birth image in the same way (see Chapter Four).

The first 15 to 20 minutes of the CD cover pregnancy. So in the early stages you can listen to just this first section of the CD, and bring yourself out of hypnosis before the part for the birth. At the start of this section I say, "And now in a few weeks your baby is going to be born so easily, naturally, comfortably."

To take yourself out of hypnosis, all you have to do is to open your eyes and count 1, 2, 3, 4, 5 (either silently to yourself or out loud). This is also stated at the start of the CD, so it becomes a trigger for your unconscious mind. You can do this if you are disturbed when listening to the CD (for example, if the telephone rings and you feel you need to answer it), or to come out of hypnosis after the pregnancy section.

I suggest you listen to the entire CD several times before you concentrate on the pregnancy part, so you are familiar with the whole recording. You will notice that to bring you out of hypnosis at the end of the CD, I count from 1 to 5 (this is the trigger to exit hypnosis).

Once a week listen to all of the CD.

Six weeks before your due date listen to the CD every day in its entirety.

The purpose of the CD is to help you through your pregnancy so you enjoy it; so you are relaxed and in control at the three stages of birth, coping easily with the contractions; so you bond with your baby and breastfeed easily; so you can get your figure back to pre-pregnancy size, shape and weight quickly after the birth; and so you can become a natural earth mother.

The CD has a trigger (which you can say out loud, or silently to yourself) so you reinforce the entire hypnotic programme with your conscious mind. The trigger is "wonderful childbirth".

The main purpose of the CD is to help you deal with the contractions. As I explained in Chapter Six, the uterus is made up of smooth, involuntary muscle and so is not under conscious control. Thus when you start the birth process this muscle will contract whether you want it to or not. There is nothing that you can do to stop the process. By contracting the skeletal muscles, those that move your bones, and which are under your conscious control, you simply slow down the process and often create the panic response described in Chapter Five.

Everyone deals with pain differently. When you experience pain you still have the actual organic pain itself, but you also have your psychological awareness of that pain (which is your pain threshold), and you have your own reaction to the pain (which is how much you think it will hurt). So because most mothers-to-be are repeatedly told that giving birth is painful and that the contractions are unbearable, they come to believe this.

I feel it is important, therefore, to think of the contractions as just what they are, contractions creating a pressure to help your baby out into the world. If you think of the contractions as 'pains' then 'pain' is what you will get.

So come to admire the female body and how wonderful it is in creating a new life and how amazing the birth process is, so the baby is born easily and naturally.

I have to admit that for me feeling the first very strong contraction with my first son has been the most exciting experience of my entire life, even better than the parachute jump I did to celebrate my sixtieth birthday. Being a biologist, I was very aware of how my body works and to feel that pressure, and knowing that I could do nothing about it, was incredible. So I had the choice of either working with the contractions or against them and, of course, I chose the former.

Hypnosis helps you to limit the pain to just the actual organic feelings of the contractions. By doing this you can then cut down on your psychological awareness and personality reaction to the pain by minimising your response to it. This is hypnotic anaesthesia.

There are several levels of pain control. The first level of pain control is removing the biggest obstacle, which is your fear, and so removing the panic response.

After all women's bodies are designed to give birth to babies and so it is a natural process.

The second level of pain control is created by generating a trust and belief in the hypnotic process and knowing that your body can create its own epidural by secreting endorphins (serotonins) which are similar to morphine in their effect.

Once your mind has been freed from fear and understands the working of the female body and the process of birth, then the third level of pain control is the ability to focus on your experience in the present moment and to engage in the use of progressive relaxation. Relaxation is the most important key to pain control and thus seeing the contractions as just a feeling of pressure.

The fourth level is the complete removal of the feeling of the contractions (pain) by the process of dissociation, which is achieved by self-hypnosis. With practice everyone can learn to do this. To enter a deep trance state you must be completely relaxed and rested enough to remain awake. The key is to know that you are removing yourself from the feeling of the contractions and not vice versa.

Visualisation is so important, since creating vivid memories and fixating attention on special places or relaxing colours can help you to anaesthetise any part of the body you wish. Once you are mentally detached from the contractions, it can help you towards a drug-free, painless childbirth.

Fig 8.1 The perfect contraction

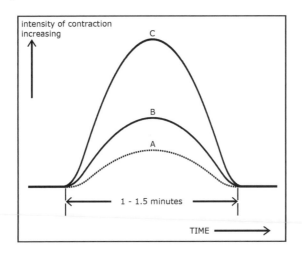

Curve A represents small, weak contractions.

Curves B to C show the contractions gradually increasing in intensity, i.e. becoming stronger.

Curve C represents the strongest contractions (occurring towards the end of phase one of the birth process and two to three minutes apart).

How you can use your hypnosis for the three stages of birth will be explained in Chapter Twelve.

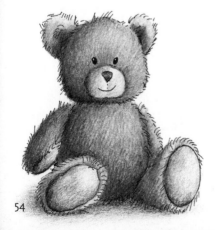

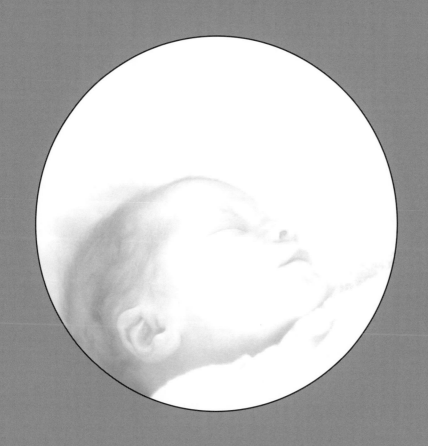

CHAPTER NINE:
GETTING READY FOR THE BIRTH

It is important to start listening to the CD as soon as you can. In this way your unconscious mind is familiar with what it has to do. Thus you are programming yourself to have the birth you desire. Then, when you have your first contraction, or the waters break, this is the signal for the entire programme to commence and so all stages of the birth simply flow.

By listening to the CD you are practising your visualisations and your colours.

At 36 weeks, you can prepare the uterus, your nipples and the perineum for the birth.

Getting the uterus ready for the birth

1. Eat fresh pineapple regularly. I suggest you eat this three to four times a week. It is an acid food and may upset your digestive system if you eat too much of it.

2. Take raspberry leaf. This can be taken as a tea or, as it is an acquired taste, it can be taken in tablet or liquid form also. Put 15 to 20 drops of the liquid (depending on the make) in a little water and drink.

Start with one cup of tea a day, one tablet or 15 drops in water, and build up gradually to a maximum of four cups of tea, tablets or sets of drops daily. The tea can be sipped freely during labour too. In my opinion the liquid method is the best way to ensure you get the correct standard dosage and it is also easily absorbed into the body. Raspberry leaf in all the forms described can be bought from a health shop.

Both pineapple and raspberry leaf contain a uterine tonic and so help to prepare the uterine muscles for the birth.

Pineapple contains the enzyme bromelain, which is thought to help soften the cervix and bring on labour. Eating large amounts of this fruit stimulates the gut and bowel and because they are the same type of muscle as the uterus this may cause contractions to start. That is why it is important not to eat too much of it, unless you do want the birth to begin.

Raspberry leaf contains a nourishing source of vitamins (A, B-complex, C and E), minerals (calcium, iron, magnesium, manganese and phosphorous) and fragrine, an alkaloid, which gives tone to the muscles of the pelvic region and the uterus itself. The vitamins and minerals help your immune system to be stronger, and facilitate healthy skin and bone development for the baby. The calcium is necessary in controlling nerve response during childbirth. The fragrine allows the uterus to contract more powerfully and effectively during labour, and if you drink the tea during the birth this will help to maintain strong contractions, so your baby is born more quickly. It allows the uterus to let go and function as it is designed to.

The high vitamin and mineral content help to replace those that are lost via blood loss in delivery and the alkaloids that are present will also aid in toning the uterus after birth, allowing it to return back to its usual size more easily. This in turn means that blood loss after the birth is minimised.

Breastfeeding tips

1. To get the nipples in peak condition, if you can, when you are at home, do not wear a bra. If this is too uncomfortable, then get an old bra and cut holes for your nipples. The friction of the nipples on your clothes toughens the nipples, ready for breastfeeding.

2. Use a nipple cream just before the birth to keep the nipples supple. In this way the nipples do not dry out so easily due to the suckling of the baby.

There is usually no medical reason why a mother should not feed her child for as long as she and the child want. Breastfeeding is a personal decision and it is up to the mother to decide what is best for her. However, it has been shown that to breastfeed for even just a few days is really beneficial to the baby. I give the reasons for this below.

The initial milk, known as colostrum, is produced for the first three days and contains protein (four times as much as ordinary milk), lactose, vitamins, white blood cells, serum and protective antibodies. Although it has a yellow colour, there is little or no fat present. It also contains a natural laxative to rid the gut of the meconium, which filled the digestive system of the baby when it was in the uterus. This natural laxative is not found in the powdered milk available, nor are the white blood cells and antibodies, which help to boost the baby's immune system.

Normal breast milk is a more watery suspension containing fats, proteins, mineral salts (especially calcium for healthy bone development) and lactose. The powdered milks simulate this milk. Production of milk continues as long as the mother breastfeeds.

Perineal massage

The perineum is the area around the vagina between the vagina and anus. Massaging the perineum gradually softens and stretches the vagina and perineal tissue in preparation for the birth. This is especially useful for first-time mothers and women over 30.

Doing this massage will familiarise you with the feeling of the pressure and stretching of the perineum that you will feel when your baby's head is being born. Being aware of these feelings helps you to relax during the birth and to actively participate in your baby's birth.

Fig 9.1 Perineal massage

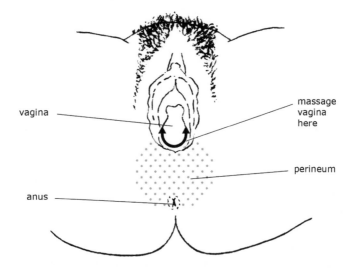

vagina

massage vagina here

perineum

anus

Either you or your partner can do this massage. Use a mirror the first few times, and look at the perineum so that you can see what you are doing. It is advisable to massage after a bath to begin with, as this will soften the surrounding tissues. Make sure you have emptied your bladder and wash your hands before you start. Find a comfortable position that works best for you. There are several positions that can be used. These are semi-sitting, reclining, squatting against a wall or standing with one foot raised and resting on the bath, toilet or chair.

The massage should be done three to four times a week for about four minutes, beginning six weeks before your due date.

Lubricate your fingers with almond oil, olive oil, or vaginal lubricating jelly (if you are sensitive to nut oils). The oil allows your fingers to move smoothly over the perineum and lower vaginal wall.

If you are doing the massage yourself, it is probably easiest to use your thumb. Your partner can use the index finger and the next finger together.

Place the fingers or thumb about 5 centimetres into the vagina. This is roughly up to the second knuckle of the fingers or thumb.

Using a sweeping motion with downward pressure, move in a rhythmic movement from side to side (as shown by the black arrow on the diagram). This movement will stretch the vaginal tissue and muscles surrounding the vagina.

You can also massage the skin of the perineum between the thumb and forefingers.

As you or your partner perform the massage, apply a steady pressure downwards towards your bottom (anus) until you feel a tingling sensation. This is similar to the sensation that you will experience when your baby's head starts to come out of your vagina. The baby is said to be 'crowning'. This massage should not be painful. If you find it painful ease off from the pressure you are applying.

Use more oil, if required, to reduce friction. Concentrate on relaxing your perineum, that is, your pelvic floor muscles.

When you start doing this massage you will feel tight, and as you continue to practise it the tissues will relax and stretch, and the massage will become more comfortable.

By doing this massage, you get the vagina and perineum used to the 'feelings' of the baby being born and so they stretch more easily, as you are much more relaxed at the birth. Many women who have done this massage regularly have found that they did not tear at the birth. Thus I would really recommend that you do this.

Pregnancy yoga

This is very beneficial at all stages of the pregnancy. It teaches you relaxation through exercise and breathing. It works really well with the hypnosis because it reinforces that you can be in control, to deal with the contractions and the birth process.

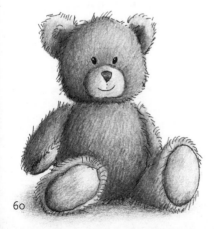

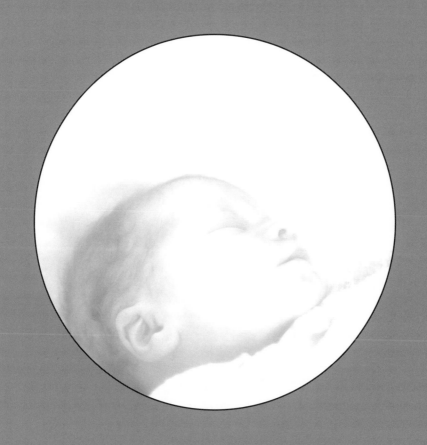

CHAPTER TEN:
WHAT TO DO IF YOU HAVE ...

Having used your CD, you are now familiar with using your colour of relaxation. You know which colour is right for you and your unconscious mind. This colour is also very powerful in healing. So use this colour to create healing and changes within yourself.

Using the programme for the three deeper breaths (described in Chapter Five) is also very beneficial in healing.

Nausea and vomiting in pregnancy

Sickness and nausea are a result of the hormone changes taking place in the body and the digestive system being more sensitive in the early stages of pregnancy. For most women, these feelings disappear by week 14.

For some pregnant women, the symptoms are worst in the early morning, hence the term 'early morning sickness', and they ease up over the day. The symptoms can strike at any time and even last all day. The intensity of the symptoms can vary from woman to woman too.

Each pregnancy is different and not every woman suffers from this nausea. With my first pregnancy I had no nausea or sickness whatsoever, and yet with my second baby I had gentle nausea until 14 weeks all day long.

To deal with the symptoms, and to even lessen the feelings, use your colour of relaxation.

If you can, take yourself to a quiet place. Imagine being in your special place and then surround yourself, and especially your digestive system, in your chosen colour of relaxation and healing. With practice, you will be able to do this even while sitting at your desk at work, or with people around you.

Feel the colour relaxing you and healing your digestive system, so it works more efficiently and effectively for you, and feels and is more and more comfortable. Say some words to yourself too. Tell your body how you want to feel.

This then ties in with the programme for the three deeper breaths. Do this as often as you can every day.

On breath three, say phrases similar to the following:

"My digestive system is more and more comfortable."
"My hormones easily and quickly adjust to the correct levels for a wonderful pregnancy."
"I cope easily with all the changes occurring in my body."
"My body is comfortable with all the changes that are occurring within it."
"I enjoy being pregnant and find any discomfort comforting."
"I love and appreciate the changes that are occurring in my body."
"I am excited about being pregnant."

You can use any words that are right for you. These phrases are positive affirmations. An affirmation is really anything you think or say to yourself. A great deal of what we normally think and say is quite negative and this has a deleterious effect on our unconscious mind. So we have to retrain our thinking and speaking into positive patterns to change our lives and how we are feeling.

Every complaint you make or negative thought you have is affirming something you think you do not want in your life. If you feel that your pregnancy is not how you want it to be, then it is almost certain that these feelings will continue until you change the way you think and talk to yourself.

The more you choose to think thoughts that make you feel good, the quicker the affirmations work. So think happy thoughts. It really is that simple. The way you think is your choice.

Notice that all affirmations are positive suggestions asking for what you want (not what you do not want) and for how you want to feel (not how you do not want to feel). Also the affirmation is said in the present tense as if it is happening now.

The only moment you ever live in is this moment, in the now. It is the only time you have any control over your life. There is a saying: "Yesterday is history, tomorrow is a mystery and today is a gift and that is why it is called the *present.*" So live your life in the present and choose to feel good in this moment, now.

The same procedures as described above are used for all the situations that may occur in pregnancy.

Acupuncture and reflexology may also help to alleviate the nausea symptoms of early pregnancy.

Needle, doctor and hospital phobias

When you dissociate from a situation you cannot feel fear. So when you are going to the hospital or doctor, imagine you are in your special place. Really be there and see what you see, feel what you feel and hear what you hear. Also use breathing technique one, of breathing in to a count of four and out to a count of six (as described in Chapter Five), to keep your adrenalin levels low. You can surround yourself with your colour of relaxation and healing also.

Continue to do this in the waiting room and when you go into the room for a scan, blood test or any examination. Remember, having a baby is an exciting adventure and so going to the doctor or hospital for a baby is a happy thing, and quite different from going to these places because you are unwell.

Remember that you can choose how you want to feel. To reinforce this, use the programme for the three deeper breaths, creating positive affirmations at breath three. Do this daily and as many times as is possible.

On breath three say phrases similar to the following:

"I am happy to have a scan so I can see my baby."
"I am really excited about my scan and seeing my baby and maybe even finding out if it is a girl or boy."
"The maternity ward of a hospital is a good place to be."
"I sit in the waiting room and feel, and am, so calm, relaxed and in control."
"I find having a blood test easier and easier."
"Every time I have a blood test my confidence increases so each time I have a blood test it is easier and easier."
"I am calm and in control when the nurse puts the pressure band around my arm."
"I look away at this point and take myself to my special place."
"I hardly notice the needle going into my arm because I am so calm and relaxed."
"I am more and more comfortable when having an injection."
"Every time I have an injection my confidence increases, so each time I have an injection it is easier and easier."
"Every time I visit the doctor or go to the hospital my confidence increases, so each time I visit the doctor or go to the hospital it is easier and easier."
"I see things in their true perspective."

Again use any words or phrases that are right for you. Use words that entice, seduce, encourage, reassure and excite you, to make the changes you desire.

Swollen extremities

This is known as oedema (or edema) and is caused by a build-up of fluid in the tissues which has not returned to the veins to be taken back to the heart. This is as a result of the growing uterus putting pressure on the pelvic veins and the vena cava (a large vein that carries blood back to the heart from the lower limbs). The pressure slows the return of the blood from the legs, causing it to accumulate, which forces the fluid from the blood vessels to ooze out into the tissues of the feet and ankles.

Oedema is often worse in the last stages of the pregnancy, when the uterus has reached its largest size and the baby is growing rapidly, creating more pressure on the blood vessels. It can get worse in hot weather too. You may also have some mild swelling in your hands as well as the feet and ankles.

You can help relieve the increased pressure on your veins by lying on your side. Since the vena cava is on the right side of your body, left-sided rest works best. Sitting with your feet elevated above your bottom also helps the tissue fluid to drain back into the veins and back up the legs.

After you have your baby, the swelling will disappear fairly rapidly as your body eliminates the excess fluid much more easily.

Again, your colour of healing can be used to improve this situation. Surround yourself with your colour and focus it on your blood vessels. Visualise your blood system working efficiently and effectively for you, and see all the tissue fluid going back into the veins. Do this whenever you think about it, and especially at night before you fall asleep.

The programme for the three deeper breaths can also be used. At breath three, say something similar to the suggestions below:

"My blood system works more and more effectively for me."
"The tissue fluid easily and effortlessly drains back into the veins for transport to the heart."
"My ankles and feet (and hands) are more and more comfortable."

Placenta previa

Placenta previa simply means that your placenta is lying unusually low in your uterus, next to or covering your cervix. The placenta is the organ, normally located near the top of the uterus, that supplies your baby with nutrients, and gets rid of the baby's waste materials, through the umbilical cord.

If the placenta covers the cervix completely, it is called a complete or total previa. If it is right on the border of the cervix, it is called a marginal previa. (This may also be known as 'partial previa', which refers to a placenta that covers part of the cervical opening once the cervix starts to dilate.) If the edge of the placenta is within 2 centimetres of the cervix but not bordering it, it's called a low-lying placenta. The location of your placenta is always checked during your mid-pregnancy ultrasound examination. If the placenta is low it will be rechecked by another scan at 32 weeks. Most of the time it moves up in any case as the uterus grows.

The placenta (due to the way it embeds in the endometrium of the uterus) is not a fixed structure. So using your powers of healing, your body and your own self-hypnosis, you can move the placenta to a safer position for birth if you are diagnosed with marginal previa. Total previa is harder to shift in the later stages of pregnancy, due to the weight of the baby pushing down on the placenta.

To move the placenta, use your colour of healing and relaxation and the programme for the three deeper breaths again.

When you go to bed at night, before you fall asleep, surround your uterus with your colour of healing and visualise it literally moving the placenta to the 'normal' position (as shown in the diagram). Moving the placenta is usually a straightforward task unless you have complete placenta previa. However, I would still use all the suggestions given here, as even this type may be moved.

At breath three of the breathing programme, say the following:

> "My placenta glides to a safe position for my baby's birth."
> "My placenta moves easily and efficiently to a safe place so my baby is born naturally and easily."
> "My placenta moves away from the cervix because it can do so and so it does."

I would advise you to do the breathing affirmations at the same time as visualising your colour moving the placenta. Apart from one complete placenta previa, all the mothers that I have worked with have been able to successfully move their placenta to a safe place for a natural birth.

Fig 10.1 Placenta positions

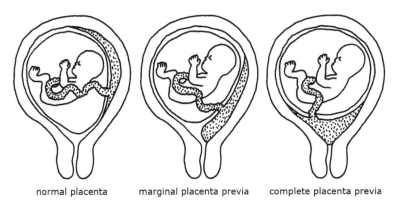

normal placenta   marginal placenta previa   complete placenta previa

Anxiety about having a large baby

Many mothers expect to have large babies when they know that they and/or their partner had a large birth weight.

You are in control of your birth. You can therefore use the inner power of your unconscious mind to control the size of your baby.

Use your healing colour to surround your baby and visualise it being the perfect weight you would like it to be, and having a wonderfully natural birth. Positive affirmations at breath three of the three deeper breaths could be:

> "My baby is a perfect size and weight for me to give birth easily and naturally and so I do."
> "My baby is ----- [give the exact birth weight you would like it to be] when it is born."

A breech baby

In the same way that the placenta can be moved, a breech baby can often be turned.

Babies move a great deal at night and so again use this process at bedtime before you go to sleep.

Surround your baby with your healing colour and visualise your baby turning to the head down position ready for birth. Use your imagination as much as you can to turn your baby. Pat your baby and talk to it. Ask it, and even tell it, to turn, as the birth experience will be so much better if it does so.

At the same time, use your three deeper breaths programme and on breath three say:

> "My baby easily turns round to the correct position."
> "My baby is in the correct position, head down, for the birth."
> "I enjoy a wonderfully natural birth."

I saw one mother who had already had a C-section, as her first baby was breech. She knew her second baby was breech also and was having a scan, two days after we met, to see if it was still breech, and to book a date for the C-section. She was uncertain about whether she wanted me to do any work in turning the baby because she was happy to have another C-section, since she knew what to expect. After we chatted a little she decided to give it a go. I gave her the suggestions above and got her to repeat this each night. After her scan, she informed me that the baby had indeed turned and how the hospital were amazed, as she was having a big baby and only had three weeks to her due date. This mother was thrilled, as she was able to experience a natural birth.

Another mother I saw was actually woken in the night by the sensations of her baby turning, and the next scan verified it had done so.

Reflexology and homeopathy can be very helpful in turning babies. Many reflexologists and homeopaths give support throughout the entire pregnancy.

Anxiety about bonding with your baby

Some first time mothers are concerned they may not bond with their baby. Be assured that this is a very common feeling. Your baby actually starts to bond with you during the pregnancy stage. Your baby can hear sounds, and feel vibrations outside the uterus, and so will be familiar with your voice and that of your partner. Talk to your baby, sing to your baby and touch your baby via your abdomen in a loving way. All this will reassure your baby and familiarise it with your voice and touch. As your baby grows, you may find your baby moves in response to your attentions, so you can converse with your baby before it is born.

As soon as your baby is born, the sounds and vibrations felt in utero will still be familiar, and thus your baby will have a sense of peace. Hypnobirthing babies usually are very calm and contented babies.

After the birth, talk to your baby. Touch and caress your baby. Welcome your baby into the world. It is very helpful to have skin-to-skin contact as soon as you can after the birth, to increase bonding. This is an exciting time. The birth is over. You have your baby in your arms and enjoy this. Your baby will pick up on this. Your baby too will feel excited about being with you. Your baby will enjoy the space outside the uterus, and also the security of being held in your arms.

Bonding is covered on the CD. As you listen to the CD daily, absorb the positive suggestions. You will become more and more confident that you will bond strongly, naturally and easily, and so you do.

Every relationship between two people is different. We all have differing maternal and paternal instincts. There are no right or wrong ways to bond with your baby. Simply do what you feel intuitively is right for you.

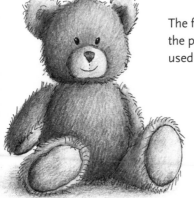

The following positive affirmations at breath three of the programme (for the three deeper breaths) can be used before and after the birth:

> "I bond with my baby naturally and easily."
> "My bond is deepening as my baby grows."
> "I enjoy talking and singing to my baby."
> "I love my baby."
> "I love touching my baby."

"I enjoy the movements of my baby as it responds to me when I talk and sing to it."
"I am excited by the feeling of my baby as it responds to me."
"It is fun being a mother and bonding with my baby."
"I am excited about meeting my baby."
"I cannot wait to meet my baby."

After the birth you can omit the last two affirmations.

Anxiety about breastfeeding

Many first-time mothers may get anxious about breastfeeding, as it will be a new experience for them. Some second-time mothers, where the breastfeeding has not gone quite to plan the first time around, may also be nervous about this with the second baby.

Many midwives and breastfeeding classes often paint a negative picture of the process. However, remember that, like birth, this is a natural process. The female body is designed to breastfeed, and most women can (unless you have a physiological problem with your breasts and/or nipples). Many women with inverted nipples can often breastfeed successfully too.

Use the programme for the three deeper breaths to boost your confidence, using the following positive affirmations at breath three:

"I breastfeed easily and naturally."
"I enjoy breastfeeding."
"I am relaxed and so my baby is relaxed during breastfeeding."
"My baby latches on so easily."
"I get my baby in just the correct position, so breastfeeding is easy."
"My baby and I both enjoy the experience of breastfeeding."
"My milk flows like a gentle stream (or fountain), so easily."
"My breasts are always comfortable while I am breastfeeding."
"My nipples are always comfortable during breastfeeding."

In Chapter Fourteen, I make suggestions as to what to do after the birth and I will cover breastfeeding in more detail. Sometimes the baby needs to learn how to latch on and, in the same way a mother needs to learn the correct position to hold her baby (to ensure that her breast and nipple are in the best position for the baby). Usually (within six weeks) any discomfort you may feel goes completely, so it is really worth persevering.

I cover breastfeeding on the CD and so, as a result of boosting your confidence, your unconscious mind then feels very happy about doing this. Usually mothers who have used the CD and followed the above affirmations are successful in achieving their goal of breastfeeding and really enjoy the experience and all the benefits it gives you and your baby.

Breastfeeding is beneficial to the baby because it is a perfect food. It also contains some of your antibodies so there is a reduced risk of your baby developing infection. It could also be beneficial to you as research is being carried out to show that breastfeeding may reduce the possibility of breast cancer, ovarian cancer, type 2 diabetes and postnatal depression. It helps you reduce your weight back to pre-pregnancy size and it is cheaper than powdered milk because it is free.

A C-section

Sometimes things happen that cannot be avoided and so if you know you are going to need a C-section then it is best to be prepared.

Again, using positive affirmations, you can help yourself enjoy the birth. These days you are usually still involved in the birth, in that you are often given a spinal block or an epidural.

The following suggestions and affirmations may be helpful:

"I am mentally calm and relaxed when I am given the spinal block or epidural, as I take myself to my special place."
"I surround myself and my baby in my healing colour during the entire procedure, so it is a calm experience for everyone."
"I enjoy talking to everyone in the operating theatre."
"My C-section is a happy experience for all concerned."
"I feel great joy as my baby is delivered by the surgeon."
"I am very calm and relaxed as my body is repaired (stitched up)."
"I trust in the healing power of my body, so the wound heals up powerfully and gently, and at a rate that is correct for my body."

All affirmations given in this section are suggestions for you to use. Please feel free to modify them to suit the words that you would normally use to speak to yourself. Simply remember to make the affirmation in the present tense, and in as positive a way as you can, always asking for what you want to happen.

Positive affirmations can be used in any situation and not just for your pregnancy and birth. Use them to achieve whatever it is you wish to improve in your life. This is a life-long skill that can be used at any time and anywhere.

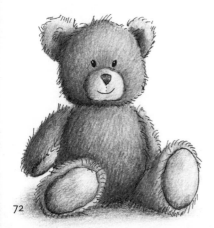

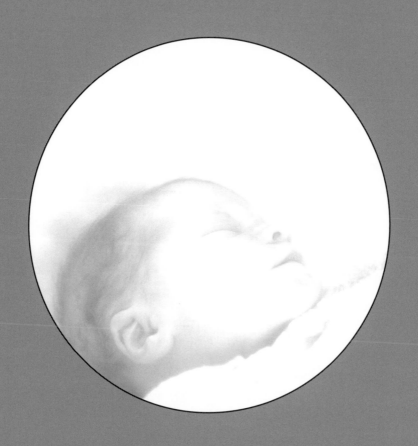

CHAPTER ELEVEN:
WHAT TO DO IF YOU GO
PAST YOUR DUE DATE

Only 5 per cent of babies arrive on the due date. The gestation period for 95 per cent of normal babies is between 265 and 300 days. The average is 282 (40 weeks), which is taken to estimate the due date. It is important to remember that some mothers just do take longer to make a baby!

Things to do when past your due date

Keep relaxed and do any of the following suggestions that feel right for you.

1. Visualisation
Use your birth image. Imagine that your baby is ready to be born and see your body start to open up naturally. Visualise your perfect birth happening now.

2. Your colour of relaxation and healing
Surround yourself in your colour to release any lingering fears, emotions, or unresolved issues that you need to release. Locked-up emotions can make you feel uptight, and cause your body to produce the inhibiting hormone catecholamine. Your tension can translate into a tense cervix, preventing the flow of your natural relaxants. Allow the colour to flow inside you, releasing any tension and calming you ready for the birth.

3. Three deeper breaths
Use positive affirmations to convince you and the baby that the time is right for your baby to be born. Say the following at breath three:

> "I am ready for my baby to be born."
> "It is OK now, baby, [or use the pet name you are calling the baby] for you to come out into the world."
> "I am really looking forward to meeting you."

One of my clients was determined that her baby was going to be born on May the 5th. So we used all the above three methods. She visualised that her baby was born on May the 5th and used her colour to ensure that her baby had completed his development by this date. She affirmed it consciously using her programme for the three deeper breaths. In fact, she started labour on May the 3rd and all was going really well. She was very disappointed about this. However, after several hours all the contractions stopped completely. It was deemed to be a false alarm. She started in earnest again the evening of May the 4th, and her baby was born at 3.00am on May the 5th as planned! This just reinforces the power of the unconscious mind and how we can determine what happens. This is the mind-body control we all have.

4. Hot and spicy foods
These can stir up the digestive system to induce labour.

5. Cleanse the bowel
Often the pulsating effect of emptying the bowel can stimulate the production of prostaglandin, the hormone-like substance that thins the cervix. Take half a tablespoon of castor oil, for three doses. (This is more palatable if followed by an orange juice chaser.) Another recipe is 25mls mixed with freshly squeezed lemon or lime juice. As the oil creates peristalsis in the bowel, it stimulates the onset of labour because the uterus also contracts by peristalsis. I took an entire bottle of castor oil in fresh orange juice (on the advice of my midwife) in one go, to help induce my second child, who was two weeks past my due date. It did start things going! However, not all midwives advocate the use of castor oil so do take their advice and if you choose this method be sure to drink plenty of water to avoid dehydration. If you choose this suggestion, castor oil can be bought on the Internet or from some health food shops.

6. Evening primrose oil
Primrose oil is rich in Omega-3 and is an excellent supplement to take on a regular basis through your pregnancy. Primrose oil can assist in naturally ripening the cervix. So start by taking two capsules orally each day, four weeks before your due date. Two weeks prior to the due date, you may insert liquid evening primrose oil into your vagina. Each evening, at bedtime, prick one end of two capsules with a pin and allow the contents of the capsules to melt in your vagina nightly, until the birth process starts.

7. Foreplay
This can trigger the hormonal connection between breast and vagina (especially stimulating the nipples and clitoris), producing the hormone oxytocin which starts uterine contractions.

8. Sex
This releases prostaglandins which help with the ripening and softening of the cervix and may break the waters.

9. A medium-hot bath

This causes relaxation. Your partner can scoop water over your nipples and abdomen, which triggers the hormonal connection between breast and vagina in the same way as love-making, producing prostaglandins and possibly the hormone oxytocin which starts uterine contractions.

10. Sage

This herb taken in tincture form or as sage tea can help to start the uterine contractions. The tincture and the tea can be bought from a health food shop.

11. Walking

Brisk walking may stimulate the uterus to start contractions.

12. Acupuncture

There are meridian points in the body that an acupuncturist is able to activate for the easy and effective induction of labour. This is a relatively easy procedure and can offer a smooth entry into birth. It is important that these points are not stimulated during pregnancy, except for the purpose of induction.

When you have exhausted all these means of natural initiation of labour, and it is determined that artificial induction by Syntocinon (synthetic oxytocin) is an absolute necessity, you still may request that only a minimal dose be administered and that it be withdrawn as soon as your body takes over. You will also want to ask that the Syntocinon dosage is not increased without your consent. Usually induction starts with a vaginal gel of synthetic prostaglandins, called Prostin, in the form of a pessary placed on the cervix. If this does not start the contractions then a Syntocinon drip is administered.

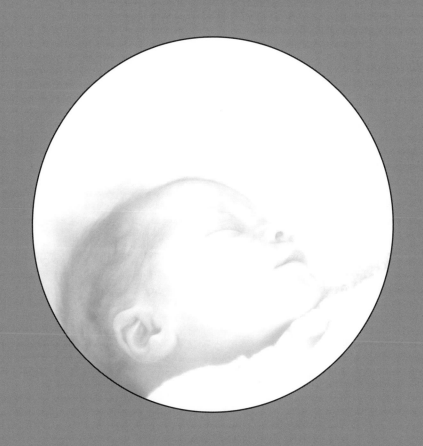

CHAPTER TWELVE:
HOW TO USE HYPNOSIS FOR
THE THREE STAGES OF BIRTH

Stage one

You are in control of your baby's birth, and if you think 'pain', then that is what you will get. You can enjoy the feeling of birth by 'tuning in' to your mind-body control, to make giving birth a magical experience, as it should be.

There are four levels of pain control.

1. The first level of pain control is to remove your biggest obstacle: FEAR. Your intellect begins to imagine all sorts of things that could happen, but fear of these inhibits two important abilities we have, of concentration and relaxation. Fear then becomes pain. The fears usually associated with pain are the fear of making it worse, fear of the unknown and what is going to happen, or fear of a past difficult birth and fear of unending pain. It is good to remember that birth does come to an end when the baby is born. The feeling of the contractions is only temporary.

2. The second level of pain control is generated by trust and belief in the hypnotic process and in the ability of your body to deal with the contractions. Remember that your body makes its own pain-killing drugs (its own epidural) by the release of serotonins. These are released in a very site-specific way in the brain, so that all the other vital systems and functions of the body continue. This is how nature manages pain control. Have you ever noticed a bruise on yourself and cannot remember how it happened?

3. The third level of pain control is to engage in the use of progressive relaxation. Once your brain has been freed from fear, you can focus your intellect and concentration on the present moment. Remember that your body is designed to give birth easily and effectively. Feel the contractions as just a pressure, instead of pain. Relaxation is the most important key to successful pain control.

4. The fourth level of pain control is dissociation through self-hypnosis. You have been practising this on a daily basis by listening to the CD.

In hypnosis you are in the alpha-theta brainwave pattern, with an altered sense of awareness. When like this, your unconscious mind cannot tell the difference between what is real and unreal. So in hypnosis you are relaxed and in control, and you allow your body to work as it is designed to do, without interference from your skeletal muscles contracting. With hypnosis, your body opens up quickly and easily. In this way, the cervix dilates to 10 centimetres quickly, and so stage one of the birth process occurs in a shorter time.

In the graph in Chapter Eight (representing the perfect contraction), the contractions for the early part of stage one are as shown on curve A. At this stage, you can simply use the breathing techniques (described in Chapter Five) and your visualisation of your special place. You can even listen to the CD. In this way you can maintain control until your partner arrives.

At this early stage you can also keep repeating the natural birth trigger for the CD "wonderful childbirth".

As the contractions move into curve B and then curve C, getting stronger and stronger, then you can use any of the techniques described below (and in Chapter Thirteen) to dissociate from the contractions. When you are in the alpha-theta brainwave pattern of hypnosis (which is also called REM: rapid eye movement sleep), this cuts out all sensory information, and in fact alters the physiology of the body, so you do not feel pain.

By using the CD, you will have been practising visualisation for the perfect birth. There is a saying, "visualise it, materialise it", and so when your first contraction starts, or your waters break, your body will be patterned to go into auto-pilot for the perfect birth.

Basically, all you need to do is to maintain a state of relaxation, and then the birth process just flows.

The CD is like installing a program into a computer. In this case it is installed into your unconscious mind and is triggered by the start of the birth process, rather like hitting the play button. So, once the birth has started and you are having regular contractions, you do not listen to the CD. Now you use all the techniques you have learnt in order to have a wonderfully natural childbirth.

Your partner is extremely important in the birthing process. Your partner's role is to talk to you non-stop for the one to one-and-a-half minutes of each contraction. This will help you remain in hypnosis, keeping you totally dissociated from your body and the feelings of the contractions. You are in an altered state of awareness and in another place of your imagination. This focused attention creates dissociation, so you are almost outside of your body.

Your partner can listen to the CD a few times to familiarise themselves with being in hypnosis. Your partner can also decide on a unique special place and colour of relaxation. They then understand what they have to do to help the hypnosis state.

If your partner feels you are losing control at any point, they can get you back into control by using either of the breathing techniques to lower the adrenalin and increase the serotonins. It is important for your partner to reassure you at all times and to tell you how wonderfully well you are doing.

Your partner can describe your special place in detail, allowing you to imagine really being there; they need to describe what you can see, hear and feel. Your partner can also use your colour of relaxation; they can tell you to imagine the colour flowing over you, like a magical shower, bringing relaxation and feelings of energy and power for a wonderful birth.

On the CD, I mention that you can use your colour as a protective bubble, which keeps out all negativity, and only allows positive thoughts and feelings to enter. So use your protective bubble to keep you safe, powerful, strong and in control throughout the birth. Use it to maintain your energy levels as well.

To help you get to the alpha-theta brainwave pattern of hypnosis more quickly, you may like to use this simple technique. It is called the 'tip-of-the-tongue' trigger. All you do is to place the tip of your tongue on the roof of your mouth directly behind your two front teeth. This little trigger can act as an anchor, and strengthen the quality of your alpha-theta brainwaves, so deepening your hypnosis.

You can say to yourself (in the early stages of the first phase curve A on the graph in Chapter Eight):

"Relax, calm, numb, courage. With each contraction, I relax more and more, and make all the muscles of my bottom nice and numb, loose and relaxed."

As the contractions increase into curve B, then your partner can say to you:

"Relax, calm, numb, courage. With each contraction, you relax more and more, and make all the muscles of your bottom nice and numb, loose and relaxed."

This is stated on the CD a couple of times, and so acts as a trigger for all the other suggestions on the CD too.

As the contractions continue to increase in power, your partner can also describe your birth image. With each breath you take, you imagine yourself stretching and opening up so easily, naturally. In this way you work with your body, allowing the natural birth process to occur. You are in control of your baby's birth.

As the contractions become more regular it is important for you and your partner to work out what is going to work best for you. So play around with all the visualisations and breathing techniques, and maybe use some of the extra ones given in Chapter Thirteen to dissociate fully from the contractions. I suggest you do this when the contractions are around 15 minutes apart.

You may find that one or two of them work best for you, so that is all you need to use. When I attended a birth with one of my hypnobirthing mums, all she wanted to do was to be on her favourite beach. As I had not been to her particular beach, I simply suggested all the usual things I knew about a beach and the sounds, feelings and sights, describing them at length. In this way, as the contractions got closer together, I was creating a wonderful picture in my mind and in hers.

Another client preferred the use of her colour and deep breathing. Work with what works best for you. There are no right or wrong ways here.

It is at this stage you can also practise using the TENS (transcutaneous electrical nerve stimulation) machine, if you are going to use this. Pregnant women and professional midwives worldwide have used this unit successfully for many years to help with the contractions. This machine can be used at home and in hospital. It can be hired from various places too, which saves you the expense of buying one.

At the onset of the birth four pads are applied to the back and the TENS unit is switched on. You feel a pleasant pulsing sensation. This helps to raise the levels of the endorphins (or serotonins), the natural pain relief chemical in the body, keeping you in control of the birth. It is important to play around with the positioning of the pads so they are placed where you actually feel the contractions.

During this first phase it is very helpful to be as upright as you can. Being upright during this stage could mean that you are standing, sitting, squatting or kneeling over a birthing ball or simply walking around.

The advantages of being upright are that you are using gravity to help you give birth, so your baby can move down more easily and more quickly. Being upright will aid dilation too as there will be more pressure from the head of the baby on the cervix.

or the first stage is to use any of the following:

* the trigger 'wonderful childbirth'
* breathing techniques
* your special place
★ your colour of relaxation
★ your birth imagery
★ any of the suggestions in Chapter Thirteen

Stage two

At the end of stage one, you will have reached contractions as in curve C of the graph in Chapter Eight. The contractions will be about two to three minutes apart. You will be in deep hypnosis now, almost permanently, relaxed and in control, feeling the contractions as strong pressure.

Sometimes a 'Transitional' phase occurs before stage two actually starts. The contractions may even pause for a time so you can simply rest for a while. For this reason this phase is often referred to as the 'rest and be grateful' phase!

Stage two starts as you notice the contractions change. You now get a very strong urge to 'bear down' and push your baby out.

The midwife may examine you to check your cervix is 10 centimetres dilated. Once this is so, you now no longer need to use the hypnotic visualisations. You will continue to be in a very relaxed state. However, at this time you really need to work with these contractions and use all your skeletal muscles, of your tummy, buttocks and thighs, to literally help push the baby along the vagina and out into the world. This stage does consume a great deal of energy.

Your partner is again very important in helping you to keep pushing. Your partner is important to keep you focused on what is going on in your body. This is the time to really work with your body and to follow the intuition of your unconscious mind. The mind-body connection is very important at this point. Be in tune with what your body is telling you. The body will signal to you to push because the urge is so strong and this is usually at curve C of the graph in Chapter Eight. The role of your partner is to tell you that you are doing a wonderful job. This is the time when you need to feel as if you are doing a poo the size of a melon. If you get the pushing correct, then these contractions are painless, even though they are the strongest ones. This is because all your energy is going into the pushing and so you do not 'feel' the contraction in the same way. (I indeed found this stage painless.)

However, it can take a few contractions to get used to that feeling. Just keep calm and work with your body, and you will get it right. You start to feel the baby as a bulge in the birth canal. Imagine pushing this bulge forward. It is an incredible feeling to feel the baby's head moving along the vagina, and also very exciting.

If you are not quite at the 10 centimetres dilation stage, you will not be allowed to push, so you have to do something completely different, while remaining in hypnosis and using the imagery that works best for you. Use the special breathing technique described in Chapter Seven. Pant, like a dog, with the mouth open, breathing in and out through the mouth, with the tongue resting on the lower lip. Continue doing this for the one to one-and-a-half minutes of the contraction. In this way, the pushing urge is abated. Lying on the left side is often beneficial to get rid of the last lip of the cervix. Very soon you will pass into the pushing stage (as described above).

At some point you will hear the midwife say that the head has 'crowned'. This is the point when the baby's head is just coming out of the vagina. This is a wonderful time, as you know you are almost there. A few more contractions and the head is out. The baby's head turns naturally, and with one final contraction the baby is born.

Your baby will still be attached to you by the umbilical cord. Hold your baby as soon as you can. This is also a good time to give your baby a first breastfeed, if your baby wants to suckle and is not too tired after the birth (if you are choosing to breastfeed). The sheer joy of holding your baby will make all the effort of the last few hours worthwhile.

Stage three

This stage often occurs without your even being aware of it. You will now be fully alert and awake and no longer needing to remain in hypnosis. However, holding your baby and talking to your partner will keep you in natural hypnosis.

While you are looking at your wonderful baby, the placenta will separate from the uterus. It is at this stage that you can choose whether to have the hormonal injection or to let nature take its course.

The contractions now stop for a while and usually one gentle contraction delivers the placenta. You may feel it sliding out as you push with the contraction, in the same way as you did your baby. The placenta weighs about one sixth to one third of the weight of the baby and it is very soft and squidgy, and as you are already wide and stretched you may not even notice its delivery.

VBAC – Vaginal birth after a Caesarean

If you have had a C-section for your first baby there is often no reason why you cannot have a totally safe and natural birth the second time, or even the third time, around.

In the hypnosis CD there is a great deal of healing and you can use your colour of relaxation to heal your scars in the uterus and abdominal wall. Your body is strong, and many women I have worked with have had a wonderful second birth after long first births and C-sections.

When you are calm and relaxed and in control in the first two stages of the birth, using your relaxation and hypnosis techniques, you are working with your body. Your body is strong and powerful and thus a natural birth is possible for you. Go for it. The experience of feeling your baby moving along the birth canal and seeing it exit your body is such a miraculous feeling.

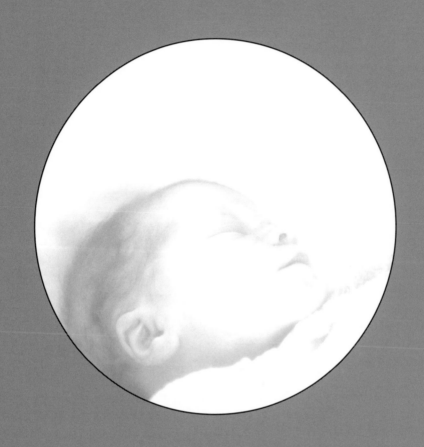

CHAPTER THIRTEEN:
OTHER SUGGESTIONS TO USE TO
DISSOCIATE YOURSELF FROM THE
FEELINGS OF THE CONTRACTIONS

Suggestions to help with the stronger contractions:

Method 1

Try to visualise the 'feeling' of the contractions as a shape. What shape is it? How big is it? Is it in more than one place?

If you were to give that 'feeling' a colour, what colour would it be? Perhaps a strong vibrant colour to match its intensity.

On a scale of 1 to 10, with 1 being low and 10 being high, where on the scale would the intensity of your feelings be? Maybe you can see a large dial, sensor, or a clock with very clear numbers on it. Now imagine the pointer at the number you gave for the intensity of the contraction. See the pointer moving backwards, so the numbers are getting lower and lower.

Think about the 'feeling' in these ways, and consciously now reduce the severity of these 'feelings'. Reduce the number on the scale down and down and down. As you do this, watch as the colour fades from a vivid shade to the palest shade possible and, as this happens, the shape becomes smaller and smaller until it is the tiniest speck.

You do not want to get rid of the 'feeling' completely, as it is there for a purpose, so you can work with your body to have a wonderfully natural birth. However, it is possible for you to manage the 'feelings' at a comfortable level.

Your partner can ask you the questions as indicated above. He can get you to visualise a dial or clock face and he can actually suggest you see the pointer moving down the numbers. He can even suggest that as the pointer moves down this anaesthetises the feeling of the contraction. As he gets to five and then four he can pause and ask – what shape is the contraction now? How big is it? What colour is it?

Method 2

When your partner touches your shoulder (or any place that you would like to be touched – it could be your arm or hand), you feel, and are, more and more relaxed and calm. And so the touch also anaesthetises the 'feeling' of the contractions.

Your partner can say, "When I touch you (or caress you) this anaesthetises the feeling of the contraction." Again, this is the mind-body connection.

The unconscious mind is so powerful it is able to anaesthetise parts of the body if it chooses to do so.

Method 3

Imagine a bowl full of hot water – just a bearable temperature for your hand. Imagine that you are placing your hand into the bowl of hot water and imagine the feeling as the heat transfers from the water to your hand, until it is full of the penetrating heat.

You can now visualise your warm hand on any part of your body, where you feel the 'feeling of the contraction'. Imagine the heat is transferred to your body and, as this happens, your body is anaesthetised by the heat. Just feel how the warmth is taking away any residual 'contraction feeling' until you feel, and are, quite comfortable.

If it is a hot day, you might prefer to imagine a bowl of cold, cool water.

Your partner can describe this situation, as if they are doing it in your imagination. (They are not really putting their hand into the water.) They can then place their 'warm' (or 'cold') hand on your body where you are actually feeling the strongest feelings for the contractions.

Again, your partner can state, "When I put my hand on your tummy (back, lower abdomen) this anaesthetises the feeling of the contraction. Feel the warmth (coolness) of my hand soothing your body and anaesthetising it." Using the imagination is a really powerful tool used to create that mind-body connection and dissociation from the contractions.

Remember, when you are in a very deep state of relaxation you do not feel fear, tension or 'pain'. So use your imagination to the very best of your ability. This really helps you to have a wonderful birth.

Remember, it is you who is giving birth and it is your baby. Your birth experience needs to match whatever is best for you and your family, and that is all that is important.

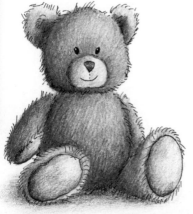

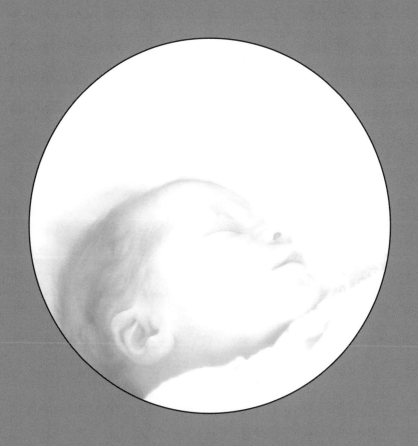

CHAPTER FOURTEEN:
THINGS TO DO AFTER
THE BIRTH

Arnica tablets

Arnica is a herbal remedy. Most people know of the cream for bruises. It is also in a homeopathic remedy form, again available from most chemists. You can consult a local homeopath to ask for advice. They may recommend that you take Arnica-30 just before the birth, when your contractions begin or your waters break, and continue taking it for a week after the birth. The usual dose is two pillules four times a day, but it can vary according to your response – if it is working well you may well need less. These little sugar balls containing the Arnica are sucked and not swallowed.

If you know you are going to have a C-section then you may be advised to start taking Arnica for two weeks before the C-section is planned (e.g. taking four pillules daily). Immediately after the birth you may be advised to take one pillule every hour for six hours, and then four daily for up to two weeks.

Glucose tablets

Giving birth is hard work. It uses up all the stored energy reserves of ATP (Adenosine Tri-Phosphate). This is stored in the muscles and liver and is made from the oxygen we breathe in and the digested food from the blood. This energy store can be remade quickly, and in order to help this process all you have to do is to eat glucose tablets in the form of dextrose. These can be bought from the chemist, as Dextrosol (Dextro Energy). Make sure to buy pure dextrose, without any additives.

Before the birth, buy 16 packets of glucose tablets, and as soon as you have given birth to your baby start munching your way through four packets a day for four days. This will mean that on day four after the birth (which coincides with the total reorganisation of the body's hormones involved in birth, and also when the later mature breast milk comes in) you are going to feel great and full of energy.

This is contrary to what most mums are told, which is that on day four they are going to feel miserable. When I had my babies, the 'baby blues' and postnatal depression (PND) were not even mentioned. This is not to say it did not occur sometimes. However, today I feel that so much is documented about this, and since the biology of birth is not fully understood by most mothers then they come to expect it. Being told it is going to happen is negative hypnosis. If you are told this often enough, then you expect it to happen and so it does happen. Again this is an example of the mind-body connection.

Therefore, when you hear this from the midwife, at the antenatal classes, or read it on the Internet, use your protective bubble of colour to reflect all this negativity, and only allow the positive feelings to enter.

Taking the glucose for a few days, and understanding why you are doing so, means that you are in control of your body and you replenish the store of ATP quickly and easily. Then, on day four, you feel wonderful, happy and excited to be a mum.

It is important to remember that only 15 per cent of mothers do suffer from PND, and many mums do not even notice the 'baby blues' because they are so happy with their baby.

Since glucose is a very small molecule it needs no further digestion. It is in fact absorbed though the lining of the mouth and will give you a quick boost of energy almost immediately. For this reason, glucose tablets can be sucked during the birth to maintain your energy levels. You might like to buy a few extra packets for the birth, too.

Please note that if you are diabetic do not take this extra glucose unless you are allowed to by your doctor.

Breastfeeding tips

When you are breastfeeding, then it is important to get your position and that of your baby correct. You will have probably been to a breastfeeding class before the birth and so you may have been shown the correct way to feed your baby.

Remember, your baby needs to get a big mouthful of breast from underneath the nipple. Place your baby with its nose level with your nipple. This will allow your baby to reach up and attach to the breast well. It is important that your baby takes in the nipple as well as the brown area of the breast known as the areola. When you do this then it is less likely that you will get sore nipples and the baby will be getting more milk.

To attach your baby to your breast, hold your baby close to you with its nose level with your nipple. Wait until your baby opens its mouth really wide with the tongue down, rather like a big yawn. You can encourage the baby to do this by gently stroking its top lip. Quickly bring your baby even closer to your breast. Your baby will tilt its head back and come to your breast chin first. In this way your baby should take a large mouthful of breast, with your nipple going towards the roof of its mouth. Your baby's chin should be touching your breast, and your baby is now latched on.

To help you get yourself and your baby in the correct position for breastfeeding you may like to consider buying a nursing or maternity pillow.

There are two things that may happen during the early stages of breastfeeding. (Note the word 'may' as this is not a certainty.) Some mothers may get sore nipples and some get a discomfort over the entire breast, which may be mastitis.

Should you get sore nipples when breastfeeding, then check the position the baby is feeding (your midwife will advise you). You can also keep some raw grated carrot in the fridge and, after feeding your baby, place some of this cold grated carrot inside your breast pad against your nipples. Not only is this very soothing, but it also encourages the nipples to heal very quickly. Another solution that is often recommended is to use mature breast milk itself as a lotion, by rubbing it into the nipple.

If your entire breast feels uncomfortable, especially when the mature milk floods in (after the four days of colostrum), or you have a touch of mastitis, consult your midwife for more advice. You can keep a savoy cabbage in the fridge. After feeding your baby put an entire leaf around each breast. Again this is very soothing and healing. Another method to bring relief is to use hot and cold flannels. Place a hot flannel – as hot as you can bear – on your breast and leave it until cooled and then replace this with a bag of frozen peas wrapped in a flannel. Repeat this three times a day.

Usually you are aware of the uterus contracting slightly while you are breastfeeding. This is quite normal and it is the uterus contracting back down to its usual size, helping you to get your figure back to its pre-pregnancy size and shape. Some mothers get very strong uterine contractions while breastfeeding, and if you find these uncomfortable, then you may be advised to take the homeopathic remedy Cimicifuga-200 to ease them. This can be bought from a good health shop.

Exercises to do after the birth

The following exercises should be repeated for six weeks (or for as long as is necessary) to help your body to return to its pre-pregnancy size, shape and weight.

Start with six to eight movements, gradually increasing. All the lying down exercises can be done on your bed.

Day 1

1. Lying with the knees bent – abdominal breathing.

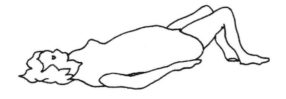

2. Lying with the legs straight – flex feet forwards and backwards to tighten and relax the leg muscles.

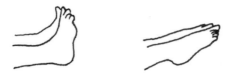

3. Lying with the knees bent – lift the head.

Day 2

1. Lying with the knees bent – tighten abdominal muscles and buttocks to press a hollow out of your back.

2. Lying with the legs crossed at ankles – contract pelvic floor muscles.

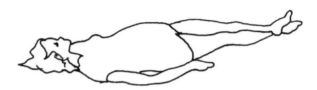

3. Lying with the knees bent – lift head and shoulders.

Day 3

1. Lying with the hands on hips – draw up one hip and push down with opposite hip.

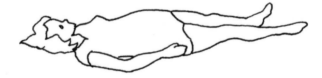

2. Lying with the knees bent – raise your head and one arm to the opposite knee, and lower. Repeat for the opposite side.

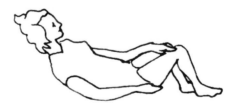

3. Standing against the wall in the correct posture.

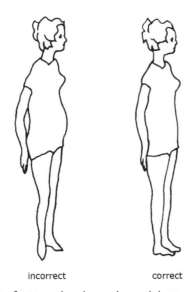

incorrect   correct

The correct posture is feet together, knees braced, bottom tucked in, tummy tucked in, shoulders straight, chin in and head up.

Day 4

1. Lying with the legs straight – raise right leg, swing over to left side of bed, raise leg to upright position, lower. Repeat with your opposite leg.

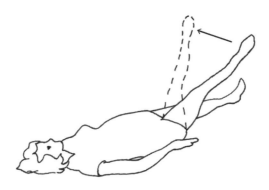

2. Kneeling on all fours – hump and hollow back.

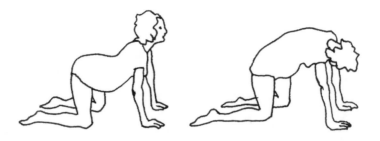

3. Standing with your legs crossed, raise up on your toes with pelvic floor contraction.

4. Lying with the knees bent – lift hips up off the bed.

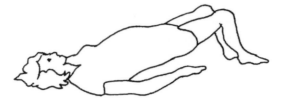

Day 5

1. Lying with the legs straight – raise your right hand to your left ankle, lower your leg and arm. Repeat with your opposite arm and leg.

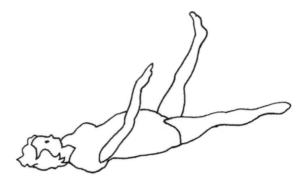

2. Standing against a wall, with your trunk dropped loosely forwards, uncurl slowly.

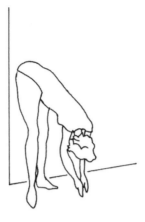

Day 6

1. Kneeling on all fours – raise your right knee to your nose, then stretch your leg backwards, lower. Repeat with other leg.

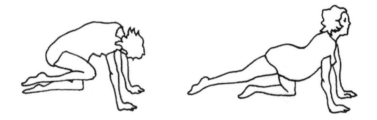

2. Lying with the knees bent on your tummy, circle the floor.

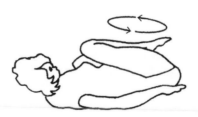

These were the exercises I did when I had my babies. I found they really helped my tummy flatten, so I was back in my pre-pregnancy clothes 10 days after each birth. Thus I really do recommend doing these exercises.

Suggested shopping list for after the birth

16 or more packets of Dextrosol
Arnica-30 (if you have taken advice on this)
Carrots
Savoy cabbage

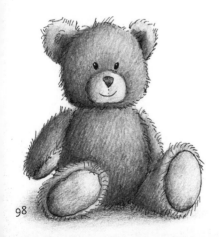

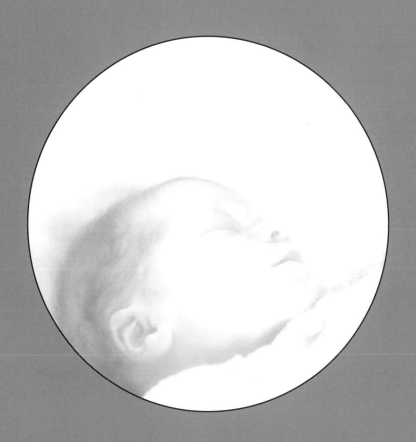

CHAPTER FIFTEEN:
ENJOYING YOUR TIME
AS A MOTHER

Now you have your baby and you are enjoying motherhood. The hypnosis and all the relaxation techniques that you have learnt from this book will remain with you for life.

You now trust your intuition and instincts. You will learn to understand your baby and its unique needs more than anyone else. You have learnt to cope with all you have to do and to have all the energy you need.

If you have other children, you know how to be calm and relaxed, coping wonderfully with all your children and your new-born infant.

Being calm and relaxed will strengthen your relationship with your partner, so you become a loving family.

Continue to use these relaxation techniques. Relax in your special place, and let your colour of relaxation flow over you. Maintain the feelings of calmness and being in control throughout your entire life.

In your imagination, use your protective colour bubble as a shield to protect yourself from negativity, from yourself and other people and anything you might hear or see or read. Feel, and be, confident in all that you do.

Use your programme for the three deeper breaths (along with positive affirmations) to keep you calm, and for whatever it is you wish to achieve, to improve skills and simply to enjoy life.

All that remains for me to do is to wish you a very enjoyable birth and happy motherhood. I hope you enjoy it all as much as I have done.

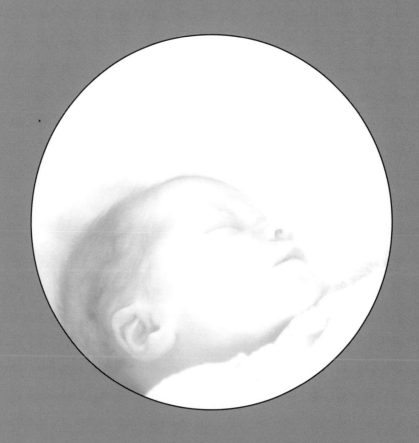

NOTES